—THE—
CBD
BIBLE

—THE—
CBD
BIBLE

Cannabis and the
Wellness Revolution
that Will Change Your Life

DR. DANI GORDON, MD

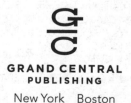

GRAND CENTRAL
PUBLISHING
New York   Boston

Grand Central Publishing
Hachette Book Group
1290 Avenue of the Americas, New York, NY 10104
grandcentralpublishing.com
twitter.com/grandcentralpub

Originally published in 2020 by Orion Spring, an imprint of the Orion Publishing Group Ltd, in London, UK
First U.S. Edition: September 2020

Grand Central Publishing is a division of Hachette Book Group, Inc. The Grand Central Publishing name and logo is a trademark of Hachette Book Group, Inc.

The publisher is not responsible for websites (or their content) that are not owned by the publisher.

The Hachette Speakers Bureau provides a wide range of authors for speaking events. To find out more, go to www.hachettespeakersbureau.com or call (866) 376-6591.

Library of Congress Cataloging-in-Publication Data

Names: Gordon, Dani, author.
Title: The CBD bible : cannabis and the wellness revolution that will change your life / Dr Dani Gordon.
Description: First U.S. edition. | New York, NY : Grand Central Publishing, [2020] | Originally published: London, UK : Onion Spring, 2020. | Includes index.
Identifiers: LCCN 2020014848 | ISBN 9781538736067 (trade paperback) | ISBN 9781538736074 (ebook)
Subjects: LCSH: Cannabinoids—Therapeutic use—Popular works. | Cannabinoids—Health aspects—Popular works. | Cannabis—Therapeutic use—Popular works. | Cannabis—Health aspects—Popular works.
Classification: LCC RM666.C266 G66 2020 | DDC 615
LC record available at https://lccn.loc.gov/2020014848

ISBN: 978-1-5387-3606-7 (trade paperback), 978-1-5387-3607-4 (ebook)

Printed in the United States of America

LSC-C

10 9 8 7 6 5 4 3 2 1

CONTENTS

INTRODUCTION

Bex came to see me for anxiety, feeling overwhelmed by the demands of her job as an advertising executive. She was having trouble sleeping, had lost her appetite and felt a constant fluttering in her chest, day and night. When we talked a little more about her symptoms, it became clear that alongside anxiety, she was also suffering from chronic stress. She used to practise yoga, but lately her anxiety had become so bad that even sitting for the 5-minute meditation at the start of the class had become intolerable, and she had given up. Her doctor had prescribed tablets, but Bex was concerned about getting hooked on them and had come to see me in search of a more natural approach. She had heard of medical cannabis, although she had never smoked a joint in her life, so she was also nervous about trying it.

I see a lot of patients like Bex in my practice, aware that something is not right but confused about where to go for help. Their doctors are often rushed and under time pressure, which makes them likely to write a prescription for antidepressants or sleeping pills. And yet when these patients look into the options for managing their symptoms naturally, there is a baffling world of pseudoscience and misinformation out there. Bex had heard anecdotally that CBD might help her, but she had no idea how to approach it, and she was worried about getting high or 'being on drugs'.

I was able to reassure her that the type of medical cannabis I would be recommending for her anxiety contained very low levels of THC, which is the compound that gets you high. She wasn't going to be taking anything that would compromise her abilities at work, change her socially or make her feel intoxicated. I put her on a very high-CBD and low-THC oil for the daytime, and at night a very tiny

1

dose of a slightly different oil with THC that would be more calming, to help her sleep.

After three months, Bex was sleeping better and had agreed with her doctor that she would come off her anxiety tablets. She told me she felt calmer, even on a stressful day at the office. We built on this success and got her back to her yoga class and working on her sleep patterns. After six months, she declared she hadn't felt this good in ten years. She claimed it was like someone had dialled back time and returned her to her old self.

Bex is just one of thousands of patients I have been able to help by using the cannabis plant as medicine to treat everything from anxiety to epilepsy. Cannabis has been used for healing over thousands of years by most of the major old-world cultures, so it's nothing new; it has just been rediscovered by modern medicine after decades of being demonised in the War on Drugs.

As a doctor, I went from being what I call a 'canna-sceptic' to being 'canna-convinced' after witnessing life-transforming results by treating my patients with medical cannabis and CBD. I have seen success after success with patients who were often at the end of their tether, having tried and been failed by countless other drugs and complementary therapies.

I consistently hear feedback such as: 'This has changed my life', 'This has saved my marriage', 'I have my life back', 'Our entire family is transformed' and 'I have rediscovered my joy for life'. These reactions have made me almost evangelical about sharing what this amazing plant has to offer us, and in The CBD Bible I have used my years of clinical practice, as well as my own personal experience, to share my knowledge of how medical cannabis and CBD can help give you a route to your best possible self.

The cannabis plant has so much to offer the ongoing wellness revolution, but there is still a great deal of confusion, conflicting information and myth surrounding it, making it hard to know what to believe. People are searching for a guide on how to safely and confidently incorporate this plant into their lives for a variety of wellness and health purposes. This book is that guide.

This is also a story about how the cannabis plant helped me, members of my family and thousands of my patients to find balance in an unbalanced modern world. It is about how this humble plant can help reclaim your inner balance, what scientists call homeostasis.

Cannabis, despite being a perfectly respectable botanical medicine, has fallen into disrepute in the last century. I am glad to see it happily regaining its rightful place as an effective and, when used properly, safe herbal medicine that has superpowers in helping with chronic symptoms and diseases, where our best modern drugs still fall short. It's not a cure for everything, but as far as tools go, it's one of the most powerful that I've ever used, in either Eastern or Western medicine.

There is no right or wrong way to use this book. If you are curious and want to know every nitty-gritty nerdy scientific detail about the cannabis plant and its compounds, then by all means read it from start to finish, including the more technical chapters in Part One about the history of the plant and the detailed ways to dose it and use it. If that seems overwhelming, don't worry – that's normal. Each of the subject/problem-focused chapters in Part Two is meant to be a stand-alone reference for you. For example, if you are most interested in improving your sleep, read the sleep chapter and then, for more detailed information about how to choose an exact product and dose it, turn to Chapter Five on dosing and how to take cannabis. In all cases, taking CBD or medical cannabis should only be considered after consulting your doctor first. No book is a substitute for individual medical advice.

Part One

CHAPTER ONE

HOW WE GOT HERE

Cannabis sativa is a plant with multiple medicinal and wellness uses. It contains hundreds of plant chemicals, including over a hundred cannabinoids that work with our bodies to help fight inflammation, protect the brain against stress, lower anxiety, impact sleep and our immune system function and may help keep us balanced, calm and happy in our hectic modern lives. I will fully introduce you to the plant and its history in Chapter Three: Meet the Plant.

CBD is one single chemical from the plant. It has many of these super-powers even on its own, and because it doesn't contain THC, it won't make you feel funny, high or intoxicated. Indeed, it is so safe that even if you swallowed an entire bottle of a hemp-based CBD oil from a health store, it probably wouldn't cause you any harm. There is a lot of fear and misinformation around the use of CBD – I have even seen someone claim to get high from a CBD facial, which would be impossible! CBD doesn't cause intoxication or make you feel high and is considered safe, especially at the average wellness doses used. According to the report on CBD by the World Health Organization (WHO), the potential toxicity of CBD was extensively researched and determined to have 'relatively low' toxicity. To my knowledge, no one has ever 'overdosed' on CBD, so it is arguably safer than many or even most over-the-counter medications for pain, cough and cold symptoms and safer than many other herbal products available at most grocery and health shops (however, always consult a doctor before starting any new supplement and see Chapter Six for those who should probably avoid CBD).

CBD can be an amazing preventative medicine tool. Thanks to its potent anti-inflammatory and stress-reducing properties, it may even help prevent health issues that arise due to unchecked chronic inflammation and stress, the perfect botanical helper for modern life.

Now cannabis is reclaiming its historic position as a part of our culture, and radically transforming everything from healthcare to the food industry and beauty products. It may even change the way we socialise, as many people are looking for alternatives to alcohol when it comes to social and stress-relief tools. Unlike alcohol, which is neurotoxic, CBD is neuroprotective (i.e. brain protective) and won't give you a nasty hangover!

What about the evidence for cannabis and CBD?

Like all herbal medicines, cannabis is tricky to study in the same way as a drug, due to the fact that it contains hundreds of plant chemicals. This is unlike pharmaceutical drugs, which are usually single chemicals with a specific target in the brain or body and dosing that follows a 'one-size-fits-all' model.

Doctors, researchers and basically everyone who reads the news have grown used to thinking that the only evidence and research that counts for a medical product is that proven using a randomised placebo-controlled trial (RCT). This model of research was originally designed for multi-billion-dollar companies to develop single-ingredient man-made drugs they could then patent, reclaiming their development costs and controlling all the conditions in a strict lab-like setting. Over the last 30 years, the drug development funnel/ RCT together became considered by definition 'evidence-based medicine', while everything else was pooh-poohed, disregarded or dismissed as lacking evidence. This agenda resulted in all plant medicines, as well as many other low-risk traditional therapies, being ignored, despite thousands of years of traditional use, doing a disservice to both patients and the pursuit of good science.

Cannabis and other botanical medicines are not as simple to analyse using the same research methods as single-chemical drugs because they contain hundreds of active compounds and come in dozens of forms. Unlike most other single-plant or man-made compounds, CBD on its own works on so many different systems and mechanisms, which accounts for why it seems to work for diverse issues, ranging from skin complaints to epilepsy.

Professor David Nutt, one of the world's foremost experts in drug effects on the brain, and a leading visionary in drug policy and neuropsychiatry, says that: 'Cannabis is arguably the world's oldest medicine, which was banned internationally for over 50 years for political reasons. I welcome its return to medical use and believe it will be the biggest innovation in new treatments in the next quarter of a century. But for patients in the UK to benefit maximally requires a change in mindset from the medical profession, who should see medical cannabis as an opportunity not a threat.'

Thankfully there is a great deal of evidence for CBD and cannabis as both wellness tools and serious medicine. This body of evidence is growing exponentially, despite the fact that it has been illegal to study the plant at all for most of the past 100 years. Considering this decades-long hiatus and the fact that plant medicines are tricky to study, we are actually moving at near warp speed when it comes to increasing the evidence for the uses of the cannabis plant.

Power plants

In herbal medicine, there are some plants I like to think of as 'power plants'. These are plants with very potent properties that can be used either for good or for bad – to heal or to harm. They are all very active, and can have strong effects even at small doses.

The main power plants that are widely used as either medicines or drugs are:

- Poppy – both morphine and heroin come from it.
- Coca – most famous as cocaine, but the people of the Andes chew unprocessed coca leaves to ease altitude sickness and help them climb up the mountainsides carrying 50 lb packs. In South America, coca leaf is also sold as a wellness tea widely used to help with focus, similar to the way we might drink a cup of coffee.

- Coffee – the morning caffeine hit that can be great in small doses for some of us, but damaging to sleep and stress in others.
- Tobacco – nicotine is one of the most addictive substances known to man, but the plant is also a powerful natural insecticide and used ceremonially in Native American traditions.
- Cannabis – one of the oldest herbal remedies, used medicinally and for spiritual purposes in many cultures over thousands of years. In modern times, the plant has been bred on the black market to create super-high-THC types for the sole purpose of getting stoned. It can also be bred for more medicinal strains higher in CBD (and low in THC) that don't tend to have this effect.

Other than poppy, which is a nervous system sedative, all the other power plants listed here, except cannabis, contain powerful stimulants. Cannabis, on the other hand, can be used to help our brain, nervous system and body return to a state of balance, harmony and equilibrium. Depending on the form and strain chosen, it can be either energising *or* calming. It has so many variations, and that's one of the things that makes it both unique and useful for many wide-ranging health uses.

Cannabis is a bridge between drugs and botanical medicine

Cannabis is being used by Western medical doctors and prescribed similarly to a mainstream drug in countries like Canada, the US and the UK alongside pharmaceutical pills. At the same time, it is still a botanical or herbal medicine – a plant medicine – with hundreds of different active chemicals all working together in harmony, unlike any synthetic drug on the planet.

The incredible thing about the cannabis plant is that it is both a botanical medicine and a drug. It can radically decrease seizures in children with drug-resistant epilepsy, with fewer side effects, and it can also change our reaction to stress and trauma.

It is also unique in that it is one of the only botanical medicines that can be used topically as acne cream and for muscle pains, taken internally by mouth, used vaginally and rectally as suppositories, inhaled via vaporising for almost immediate effect, taken 'transdermally' through the skin via a patch to affect the whole body and safely combined with many other herbs and drugs.

Cannabis also acts as a bridge between Western medicine and natural herbal medicine, bringing together people across the spectrum, from the most cynical medical doctor to the traditional medicine woman. Naturopaths and herbalists, activists, research scientists, shamans and people from all backgrounds and beliefs can talk to each other about the cannabis plant in some shape or form.

It gets sceptical people who don't believe in alternative medicines talking to people who haven't set foot in a medical establishment for years, because no matter what your beliefs, cannabis and CBD may have something to offer you. I've trained and practised for many years as both a Western medical doctor and an integrative medicine and herbal medicine specialist, and I can tell you with complete confidence, after treating thousands and thousands of patients, that this plant is special.

No other drug, herb or single ingredient I can put into a pill has the ability to bridge worlds like the cannabis plant. Many people are calling the resurgence of cannabis as a medicine and wellness tool 'the Green Revolution' and it may not be an exaggeration.

How I went from 'canna-sceptic to 'canna-convinced'

Like most people, my first exposure to cannabis was being offered high-THC joints at house parties. Many of my friends smoked weed alongside cigarettes and drinking alcohol as part of teenage experimentation. I still to this day have never smoked a cigarette and only tried cannabis for the first time when I was in my twenties – basically to see what all the hype was about. It never played a role of any sort in my life as I went through medical school, recreationally or otherwise, maybe partly because it had been drummed into me that cannabis was bad for your brain, could make you stupid or mess with academic performance.

So even though I was trained in integrative medicine (including botanical medicine!) and used other botanical medicines and natural supplements, as well as teaching my patients breathing exercises and meditation, I had quite a few hesitations about prescribing cannabis. In medical school, we were taught nothing about cannabis as a medicine, only that it was a 'dangerous' drug, despite it being available for certain medical patients legally since 2001 in Canada (a fact that no one mentioned anywhere in my training). It was as if medical cannabis was my profession's best-kept secret.

There were also the regular cautionary updates from our governing bodies about the dangers of prescribing medical cannabis and, especially in the early days, doctors were encouraged to refrain from talking about it to patients, avoid condoning it, and definitely not prescribe it. None of these warnings would ever discuss the differences between CBD and THC, or mention the research being done, unless it was a negative or poorly done study or one involving synthetic man-made cannabis products completely unlike what I would actually prescribe to someone.

Needless to say, after a lifetime of cannabis negative conditioning, I had my own prejudices against this plant to work out. Even though I was a trained natural medicine specialist doctor, I still had deeply held (subconscious, even) beliefs about CBD and medical cannabis, such as:

- Medical cannabis was just an excuse for stoners to get high legally.
- There was no 'evidence' for it working (this was what our regulatory bodies kept telling us, despite evidence to the contrary).
- It was highly addictive.
- It would increase people's risk of developing serious mental health problems.
- It can cause irreversible damage to the brain in adults.

- It was a gateway drug to addiction, ruined lives and hard drugs that destroyed a person from the inside out.
- It made people lazy.

I had seen dispensary walk-in clinics giving out cannabis and saw the issues with this model too. I knew personally some of the doctors who worked there prescribing cannabis (which was technically more like a doctor's note authorising them to use it for medical reasons vs a traditional prescription), and I felt it was done willy-nilly after a 5-minute chat, without any real understanding of the plant – dosages and different strains – or any guidance to the patient on how to use it. There was the perception that this was just an easy way for doctors to make money, writing quick prescriptions and practising bad medicine. I wanted to avoid this so, when I did start prescribing, I treated cannabis as any other integrative medicine intervention: in the context of the bigger picture and alongside other treatments. I also tweaked things like CBD and THC content, strain, dosage and method of use to suit the patient and what they wanted it for.

So what made me say yes to prescribing cannabis in the end? The first thing was my patients. I had seen first-hand patients in rural Canada growing cannabis and using it for years in place of opioids, sleeping pills and anti-anxiety medications. When they got it right, it did seem to work well. Most of them didn't smoke it, but used it in other forms like oils and vaporising. The downside of this home-grown, or 'I got it from a guy', method was the unpredictability of the result, due to not knowing what exactly they were getting in terms of CBD and THC and other plant chemical content.

I knew that by applying herbal medicine principles and a scientific method, I would be able to help make cannabis more effective and reduce the potential for any side effects or intoxication, which most people wanted to avoid. In essence, they wanted a guide they could trust, someone who understood both modern science and medicine and herbal medicine. I felt it part of my duty to help, especially since my area of interest was natural and botanical medicines. Most of the doctors prescribing cannabis, although they were doing their patients a great service in many cases, had no training in botanical medicine or deep knowledge of the plant. I was lucky enough to have been successfully incorporating these things into my mainstream medical practice for years.

The second thing that tipped me over was that I became a chronic pain patient myself after a traumatic injury and – you guessed it – cannabis helped me to heal (more on that in Chapter Twelve: Managing Pain).

So over the next few years, I devoted myself to what I started calling 'integrative cannabis medicine', and treated thousands of patients this way.

To my complete amazement, this single plant and the medicines made from it started to change my patients' lives in ways I could never have predicted. I was hearing from them on an almost daily basis that this medicine had saved their marriages, allowed them to connect with their partners, children and grandchildren or simply made them feel human again. I can honestly tell you no one had ever said that about any of the pharmaceutical drugs I had been prescribing, nor about any other single herbal remedy I had used. Something big was happening and I knew it was going to change medicine as we know it.

I'm excited to share with you in *The CBD Bible* everything I know about CBD and cannabis medicine. The plant is not a cure-all or an instant remedy for complex chronic illnesses, but it is certainly a very powerful tool to help people on many different kinds of healing journeys, and it works best alongside a holistic approach, which we will explore further in the pages that follow.

CHAPTER TWO

THE HISTORY OF CANNABIS USE

Cannabis sativa is one of the oldest cultivated plants in human history – we have evidence of likely use by humans as early as 12,000 years ago! It has been used for thousands of years for medical, spiritual and social purposes, and the fibre from the plant has been used to make clothing and rope. The seeds were eaten as a highly nutritious food long before hemp hearts could be found in the aisles at whole-food shops. It's one of the most widely utilised cultivated medicinal plants in human history across the globe. Today it's estimated that cannabis is currently consumed at least once per year, in some form, by 200–300 million people worldwide.[1]*

True plant nerds may wonder where cannabis came from. The answer from the archaeological records seems to be the Tibetan plateau in central Asia. Its closest plant relative is hops, used to make beer, and the two share some of the same plant chemicals, but it's likely that cannabis as a distinct species is at least 38 million years old. Humans evolved in places where the cannabis plant grew too, and as we will see in Chapter Four, the plant's chemical defence system is almost the perfect match for one of our own defence systems, which is why it can work in our bodies in so many ways – essentially, we evolved together.

Contrary to popular belief that until recently there was no evidence from documented medical science on cannabis, research has in fact

---

* For reference numbers indicated throughout the text as seen here, you can refer to the full list of References, which appears online at www.drdanigordon.com/cbd-bible-references.

been ongoing and documented for the past 200 years! Between 1880 and 1950, more than 30 scientific papers about the medical uses of cannabis were published, ranging from the treatment of menstrual pain and stomach ulcers to its use in severe chronic pain, insomnia and depression. This progress in publication was halted abruptly in the Prohibition era of cannabis from the mid-twentieth century until very recently, but thankfully the science and the number of research papers is catching up quite quickly.

If you want to impress your friends with your cannabis IQ, check out the highlights of the history of the cannabis plant that follow. One of the interesting things about this plant is not just how it's been used medicinally, but also how its reputation has been manipulated for political agendas, especially over the past century. In the twentieth century, thanks to the politically and financially motivated campaign against hemp and cannabis, it went from being a perfectly respectable yet potent botanical medicine to a dangerous gateway drug, in a racist and scientifically incorrect orchestrated takedown.

That may sound like a very strong statement, but it is verifiable. When I first dug into the history of cannabis and discovered its political past, my first reaction was disbelief – how could basically everything I thought I knew about cannabis and CBD be wrong? I grew up in South Carolina in the United States, and still remember the Just Say No campaign at school and the War on Drugs, both of which instilled a deep-seated fear of cannabis in me from a young age. This negative stereotype was not dispelled in medical school, where the only mention of cannabis was under the category of 'gateway drug of abuse' with no medicinal value and the potential to cause psychosis. In both the drug war and medical school, all cannabis was lumped together without any understanding of the difference between THC (the chemical responsible for the high) and CBD (which has zero chance of making you high) or the different varieties of the plant. I will get into those details in the next chapter, so hold tight for a full explanation.

Digging into the recent history of cannabis, when I first started to look into prescribing it in my medical practice, left me feeling lied to, deceived and most of all confused at how we as a culture had arrived at this demonised, unscientific view of such a useful medicinal plant. The rhetoric is still quite pervasive today, even in medical schools, but thankfully things are changing due to the recent surge in research on cannabis, CBD and the plant's medicinal benefits.

Because *any* type of cannabis use has been so vilified, often when I meet patients for the first time they confide in me that they have secretly been using it medicinally for years for various conditions. They may have started to do so as an alternative to the potentially more dangerous and addictive drugs their doctors had recommended and prescribed. They often feel a great sense of relief and catharsis to be able to tell a medical doctor what has been working so well for them for so many years without being criticised, judged or made to feel like a criminal or a lesser human. This first real conversation about the medicinal effects of cannabis with a doctor is in itself very healing. It helps the patient take control back from a medical system that has often disempowered them without offering an alternative solution. Even people who have been using mainly CBD-rich products often feel extreme guilt because it comes from *that* plant. Breaking the guilt and shame around CBD and cannabis has become one of my life's missions, because I believe plants shouldn't have morals – good or bad – attached to them.

History highlights timeline

From ancient times to the Middle Ages

Ten thousand years ago, way before the Great Pyramids were built, a human drew what appears to be a recognisable cannabis leaf on the wall of a cave in Japan on the island of Okinoshima. So it's reasonable to assume that even our cave-dwelling ancestors may have had some knowledge of the power of cannabis.

Cannabis was used in ancient Japan and China, Mesopotamia, ancient Egypt, ancient Greece, Rome and ancient India as part of both medicine and spiritual tradition. The only ancient civilisations not to use it were the New World cultures of the Incas and the Aztecs, as *Cannabis sativa* was not native to the Americas, and was only brought there by colonialism from the 1600s onwards.

Some of the first-known uses of cannabis in a major ancient culture come from China, where it was cultivated as early as 6000 BC. It was used as a medicine and for spiritual and religious purposes, as well as grown for fibre to make garments long before the hippies made hemp clothing cool.[2,3,4]

The ancient Sumerians, Akkadians and Egyptians got in on the action too, using cannabis as a medicine for problems ranging from grief to seizures and eye conditions, and even in the relief of labour pain.[5] The Romans and Persians followed suit.

However, the ancient culture with perhaps the most well-known associations with cannabis was in India. Cannabis, or *bhang*, is mentioned in the Hindu religious texts, the Vedas, as one of the five sacred plants that release us from anxiety. This long relationship with cannabis as a medicine and a spiritual tool continues even today, something I experienced first-hand on a six-month sabbatical in rural India studying yoga, meditation and Ayurveda (Indian herbal medicine) with traditional teachers. In the places I travelled to, holy towns, alcohol and meat were prohibited, but a cannabis drink called *bhang*, and *charas*, a sticky resin form, were everywhere, especially as part of the wandering ascetic culture of the *sadhus*. Followers of the god Shiva, often shown smoking cannabis, use it regularly, and share it with passers-by, who stop to sit with them. To refuse *charas* is considered rude or even unspiritual by some, so people from all walks of life can be seen sharing cannabis with one of these holy men on random street corners in many parts of India.

Interestingly, a study done on such *sadhus* living in Varanasi found that moderate long-term cannabis use in this population was not associated with any harmful effects.[6] That is not to say that there are *no* potential issues with the use of cannabis (especially high-THC, low-CBD forms, which I do not recommend for most people), but in this study, the risks appeared quite low. For the *sadhus*, it is a sacred plant, used to help attain altered states of awareness. No negative morals are attached to using it regularly for this purpose, although under current Indian and Nepalese law, cannabis use is illegal.[7,8]

Cannabis has also been used for thousands of years in the traditional Indian herbal medical system, Ayurveda, as an important ingredient in herbal concoctions made to treat conditions as diverse as fever, asthma, digestive issues, anxiety, seizures and skin disorders.[9] Without this ingredient, many of the recipes just didn't work as well – it was as though the potency had been removed from them, possibly due to the loss of synergy between cannabis and other ingredients. Ayurvedic practitioners also followed the 'less is more' approach to avoid THC overmedication and side effects, understanding that too much THC can actually cause imbalances rather than help them.

Throughout medieval Europe, the Ottoman Empire and Africa, cannabis was also widely used for a variety of purposes, including as an important medicine.

Although the cannabis plant is not native to the Americas, it was brought to the US by European explorers in the 1600s and became the most important cash crop there. In fact, in 1619 a law was passed requiring every American farmer to grow hemp, which was in some states used as a form of currency as it was so valuable.

It wasn't until 1753 that Carl Linnaeus gave cannabis the name by which we now know it: *Cannabis sativa*.

The Victorian era

The Victorians might be known for their strict morality, but they took no issue with medical use of cannabis, and there are many reports of mainstream physicians using it to treat conditions such as anxiety, insomnia and labour pains. It was available as a normal medicine in pharmacies across the British Isles and America, being used to treat everything from coughs and headaches to seizures.[10, 11, 12]

While many doctors still claim there are no Western medical publications demonstrating the use of cannabis, a study done by Dr Fronmueller in 1860 used cannabis extract to help restore better sleep cycles in 1,000 patients. There are also multiple reports of medical uses for depression and anxiety in the 1800s, including Polli in 1870 and Strange in 1883.

The age of Prohibition

This is where the confusing part begins in cannabis history, because it is filled with conflicting information and non-scientifically motivated ideas. At the very beginning of the twentieth century, things still looked pretty good for cannabis. A 1901 report by the Royal Commission concluded that it was 'relatively harmless' and not worth banning. The father of modern Western medicine, Dr William Osler, agreed and used it with good results in the treatment of migraine headache.[13] However, at the same time, doctors and governments were starting to recognise the double-edged sword of opioids (good for acute pain, bad for addiction), and they also began to realise that too much cannabis could also be detrimental, like any power plant. At the time, the cannabis tinctures available were not standardised for potency, and no one even knew what THC was yet.[14] So basically, prescribing it was a total guessing game. Many US states started to restrict access to cannabis tinctures in the same way as they were doing to opioids and medical cocaine, due to concerns over their potential dangers and misuse. This was actually a legitimate and scientific reason to monitor cannabis products that were being used as medicine. So far, so good as far as rational arguments go.

Things started to get a bit confusing and unscientific for the poor old cannabis plant around the time of the Prohibition era in the United States. There was a government-backed media and public opinion campaign against cannabis that could possibly be traced back in part to competition between hemp growers on the one hand, and cotton farmers and the timber business on the other. The theory was that hemp, as a source of fibre and possibly paper, would overtake timber and cotton, and this threatened the other industries.[15]

Another thread to the story was the fact that cannabis was widely used in African-American and Mexican social culture. The US government of the time was racist and anti-immigration, and the major newspapers created stories about 'coloured' men using drugs to corrupt and attack white women. These stories established the cannabis plant as a moral threat to society, and associated it with non-white ethnic groups.[16]

The plot thickened further after the end of Prohibition. In the midst of the Great Depression, a man named Harry J. Anslinger was appointed to form a new government department, the Federal Bureau of Narcotics (FBN). The new department needed cash and Anslinger saw an opportunity in cannabis. He is seen as the inventor of the War on Drugs in the US, and he made cannabis enemy number one.

Reefer Madness, one of the films sponsored by the FBN, can be found now on YouTube.[17] It shows people supposedly driven insane by the plant, committing heinous crimes including rape and murder. It also depicts non-white people using cannabis and corrupting white youth with it. The campaign proved very successful in creating a social and public health fear of cannabis and increasing funding for the new FBN. This set the scene for the Marihuana Tax Act of 1937, which was opposed by the American Medical Association. The Act made cannabis illegal on a federal (national) level so it became all but impossible to prescribe it as a medicine. (It is interesting to note that after the end of Prohibition, alcohol was fully rehabilitated in the eyes of American law and in Western culture. Even though alcohol is associated with many more health problems and social issues than cannabis use, it was spared the same fate.)

The next big blow for cannabis came in 1961, from an unlikely source – the United Nations.[18] Against the most up-to-date and respectable scientific research of the day, the decision was made to lump cannabis into the same danger category as narcotic drugs, opioids (such as heroin) and cocaine. This decision seems to have been based more on economics and politics than any scientific or public health reason.[19, 20] Anslinger advised the World Health Organization on the matter, leading to them saying that cannabis was considered to have 'no modern medical value'. Pretty interesting considering Anslinger was neither a scientist nor a doctor, but a lawyer and politician.

So what did the UK make of all of this? Well, a few years later, in 1968, the British government did its own homework on cannabis and concluded that 'the long-term use of cannabis in moderation has no harmful effects'. Despite this, in 1971 cannabis was removed from the *British Pharmacopoeia* and reclassified overnight to become a drug of 'no medicinal value'.[21, 22]

Thus after 1971 it was virtually impossible to study the cannabis plant for any medical purpose whatsoever in the UK or the US. And that remained the case until very recently.

Cannabis makes a comeback ...

The mid to late 1970s saw shifting attitudes towards cannabis, with the Netherlands decriminalising it. In 1988, the US Drug Enforcement Administration (DEA) ruled that cannabis clearly did have medical benefits and should be reclassified as a respectable medical drug, but this advice was ignored for another few years. In 1996, California broke new ground by making medical cannabis legal for patients with AIDS, cancer and other serious painful diseases. Finally a win for the plant!

It was the beginning of the cannabis renaissance. The EU made it legal again to grow hemp between 1993 and 1996 for most member states (very low-THC cannabis), and this stance was followed by the US in 2009. In 2001, patients in Canada got legal medical cannabis access, and in November 2018 the UK followed suit and legalised medical cannabis too.

At the time of writing, Canada and 11 US states have also legalised recreational (i.e. use without a medical prescription) cannabis for adult use,[23] and 33 states have legalised medical cannabis. In Europe, more and more countries are legalising medical cannabis, and so far the results seem overall positive, with no signs of 'reefer madness'!

Medical cannabis is even being legalised in very conservative Asian countries such as Malaysia, where a few years ago possession of a small amount of the drug could land you in jail for life.

It's quite amazing to witness this change in attitudes, and it's clear that the drive to bring cannabis back to the mainstream in a medicinal way has come from patients and advocates rather than doctors. So now you know where the plant has come from, let's take a look inside it to understand what all the fuss is about.

CHAPTER THREE

MEET THE PLANT

Remember back when you were a kid and you had to memorise plant and animal taxonomy, and how all plants and animals belong to a genus (big group) and a species (smaller group)? If not, don't sweat it, but in case you are curious, this is the breakdown of that system for the cannabis plant:

Genus (aka the wider group of plants to which cannabis belongs):
   Cannabaceae, which also contains the hop plant (used to make beer)
Species (the smaller group of specific cannabis plants): *Cannabis sativa L*
Subspecies: *Cannabis sativa ssp. indica, Cannabis sativa ssp. sativa,*
   Cannabis sativa ssp. ruderalis

Scientists are still arguing about the best way to classify the different subtypes or strains of cannabis. I'm going to simplify things to make it easy to remember and use language you will often see on labels and products in the real world to help guide you when it comes to actually choosing a CBD oil or product made from hemp that you can buy without a prescription like any other supplement, if you have legal medical access to it in your area, a medical cannabis oil or cannabis dried flower.

Trichomes: the cannabinoid factories

Trichomes are tiny sticky resinous hairs that cover the leaves and female plant flowers of the cannabis plant. They are actually a defence mechanism against insects, fungus, UV damage from the sun and animals. Plants have to have these clever defences because, unlike animals, they can't run away from danger. Instead they create a plant fortress and plan for a siege when it comes to self-preservation against any threats.

These trichomes are where the magic happens on the cannabis plant, because they produce the bulk of the cannabinoids. Creating new higher-resin (more trichomes!) varieties of hemp that are low in THC is the best way to produce CBD oil in a sustainable way in areas where it is only legal to grow hemp. The more stress the plant is under, the more cannabinoids the trichomes make in response. Often farmers will stress out the plants by changing the temperature, humidity levels, UVB exposure or the amount of light, and altering other growing conditions scientifically to get higher cannabinoid yields – which means more CBD and, if it's a higher-THC strain, more THC too.

The flowers are where most of the trichomes are, but there are smaller amounts of cannabinoids made in the leaves too.

The stalks, roots and seeds of the plant contain almost no cannabinoids.

Female vs male plants

The most concentrated source of cannabinoids (THC, CBD and the 100+ other active plant chemicals) is the unfertilised flower of the female cannabis plant, known as sinsemilla. Nowadays, cannabis that is cultivated – i.e. not wild – whether it is grown for medical purposes or recreational use, comes from the female plant. The male plants are culled to prevent the female flowers from being fertilised. That is because once the flower is fertilised, it stops making all those medicinal cannabinoids (and also the high-THC resin in the case of recreational cannabis that is grown to get you high). When you keep the female plants away from the males, it tricks the female plant into thinking it has to keep searching for a mate. So it keeps pumping out more cannabinoid-rich sticky resin to attract the male plant to come and pollinate it so it can spread its seeds (the plant version of having sex and reproducing).

Growers keep the female plants separate so they can harvest the cannabinoid-rich resin on its flowers again and again. In many cases, the female plants are now grown from a clone from one single mother plant, rather than being fertilised by a male plant. I once had a cannabis activist approach me after a lecture to share his serious concerns that this method of using the female plant and never allowing it to have sex was unethical, since it left the poor female plants forever sexually frustrated. I guess that is one way of looking at it!

The phytocannabinoids

Of the 700+ plant chemicals[1] found so far in the cannabis plant, phytocannabinoids are the group that have been the most studied so far for their effects on human health. More than 120[2] phytocannabinoid chemicals have been identified to date.

The most well-known phytocannabinoids are THC and CBD – the big two. There are, however, dozens of others that contribute to the overall health, wellness and medicinal effects of full-spectrum CBD oil and medical cannabis although we know less about them than the big two.

Cannabinoids are what we call lipophilic, which means they are fat-loving and water-hating. This basically makes them way harder to absorb when you take them orally rather than by inhalation or through the skin in a patch (like a smoking cessation nicotine patch only for CBD). However, using high-tech ways of making these products may increase the absorption by mouth too, and this area of making CBD more absorbable and more bioavailable is a whole new and exciting science in itself (see Chapter Five for more details).

I often get asked if other plants besides cannabis make phytocannabinoids, and the answer is yes! Liverwort, of the variety that grows wild in New Zealand, also produces them; one is very similar to a form of THC (called trans-THC) and is often sold as a legal-high botanical.[3] Liverwort has been used for hundreds of years as a topical medicine to help heal cuts and burns and also traditionally was used as a treatment for pulmonary tuberculosis, nerve pain (neuropathic pain) and seizures.[4] The echinacea plant (also known as purple cone-flower), used in antiviral and anti-cold botanical supplements, also makes compounds that act on the CB2 cannabinoid receptors, which interact with our immune system, one of the ways echinacea may help stave off that cold![5] The cool thing about these examples from a botanical medicine point of view is the fact that completely different plants are making similar chemicals that humans have used for thousands of years as medicines.[6, 7, 8, 9, 10]

How the cannabis plant makes cannabinoids

The 'mother' cannabinoid, called CBGA, is made first, and is then converted through a number of enzymes and pathways into the other cannabinoids, including CBD and THC.

The acid forms of both CBD and THC have an A on the end: CBDA and THCA. These are their forms in the raw plant, before it's heated up. So if you ate a raw cannabis flower or leaf, you would not get high (because THCA, unlike THC, is non-intoxicating), but the acid forms do have medicinal value too. I have patients who grow cannabis in rural parts of Canada and use the raw leaves as part of their morning green juice.

Now let's meet the most well-known phytocannabinoids, along with some of their cool but lesser-known cousins.

THC

THC is the plant chemical people first think about with cannabis, because it is the one that can make you feel intoxicated, especially at high doses in recreational cannabis strains that have been bred over the years for that very purpose. In fact, some of the lower-THC strains cultivated were named things like Hippie's Disappointment because of their lack of 'stoned' factor. Over the last 40 or so years, the recreational potency of cannabis has increased dramatically due to this desire for more and more THC. In the late 1960s, the average street cannabis might have had only around 1–3% THC, while some strains now have 20% or even higher! These 'super-potent' high-THC varieties pose additional risk in some people who may be genetically sensitive to THC, especially because they have very little CBD, which has a mitigating effect against THC's more intoxicating side effects. This is why, in general, even for medical use by prescription, it is recommended that you start with a cannabis strain low in THC and with a good amount of CBD. (For a full discussion of precautions for cannabis, see Chapter Six.)

THC locks onto special receptors in our brain and body, called the CB1 and CB2 receptors, and is considered a partial agonist of them – meaning it partly activates them. The 'high' feeling in particular comes from the effects of THC at the CB1 receptor in brain areas such as the pleasure centres, balance centres and memory centres (hippocampus), and at low doses it dampens the fear response in the amygdala. At high doses, THC can actually cause anxiety in some people (see Chapter Nine for details).

It is, however, more than just the 'high' chemical we once thought it. We now have more and more evidence of its significant medical properties too. These have been recognised since ancient times, as we saw in the timeline in Chapter Two, but modern science is finally proving these effects in animals and, very recently, in humans.

THC's medicinal properties include:

- pain relief (analgesic)
- anti-inflammatory action
- brain protection from toxins (neuroprotection)
- muscle relaxant (anti-spasmodic)
- anti-nausea
- appetite stimulant
- helps with PTSD (dampens the fear response)
- sleep promotion
- calming/relaxing (in smaller doses, usually with CBD)
- antioxidant
- anti-tumour effects (for some cancers, mainly animal models

so far; research is promising but too early to translate this into humans)
• reduces eye pressure in glaucoma

CBD

The second most common cannabinoid in the plant – and the most common non-intoxicating one – is cannabidiol, or CBD for short. Its mode of action is mainly through activating other neurotransmitter (chemical messenger) systems in the brain, body and immune system. This includes working on serotonin, vanilloid and probably dozens of other types of receptors to change chemical messages in the brain and body and influence everything from stress to inflammation and immune function.

I'm often asked about getting addicted to CBD, or having withdrawal symptoms if you stop taking it. I am glad to reassure you that this is not a risk. CBD is non-habit-forming and non-addictive – period. What I do see happen occasionally is that someone stops their CBD oil when they go overseas for a few weeks (even hemp-based CBD oils are tricky to cross borders with, so it's best not to fly with it internationally) and their anxiety or other symptoms (such as inflammation or joint pain) worsens. This is simply a return to baseline and a result of them not having the CBD in their system to effectively treat the issue. CBD, as far as we know, does not cure anxiety or pain permanently, in that if you stop taking it, the symptoms usually return. That being said, some people find that they need less of a maintenance dose of CBD for an issue like stress or anxiety once they have been stable and feeling good for a solid six-month period. This is especially true if the CBD allows them to start a meditation practice, sleep better and adopt other habits that can shift the brain out of anxiety patterns and lay down new brain networks over the top of the old anxious ones.

CBD has immense therapeutic potential and a whole host of medicinal properties in its own right. As an example, the cannabinoid pharma drug Epidiolex is virtually pure CBD and is a product that is licensed to treat certain childhood epilepsies. This CBD-only approach has advantages: it is an approved, licensed pharma drug, which is what both doctors and patients are used to; and it has to abide by incredibly high quality-control standards. However, CBD seems to work even better for some when taken alongside a small amount of THC, i.e. high-CBD medical cannabis oils and products, likely due to the synergy of the other cannabinoids. However, these full-spectrum products are harder to standardise as a one-size-fits-all drug and in some places, are not legal unless they are THC free (more on this below).

CBD's medicinal properties include:

- anti-tumour effects
- neuroprotective qualities
- analgesic properties
- anti-anxiety and antidepressant
- antipsychotic effects
- anticonvulsant (used to treat seizures)
- antioxidant
- anti-nausea (in some people works best with THC)
- anti-sebum and anti-acne effects
- counteracts THC intoxication and THC side effects (very useful where medical cannabis is prescribed for patients who may need some THC for severe symptoms but who do not want to feel intoxicated)

Other cannabinoids of interest

Other cannabinoids are found in much smaller amounts than CBD or THC in most strains of *Cannabis sativa*. However, more and more strains are being cultivated to increase the amounts of certain minor cannabinoids for their medicinal and wellness potential. It is likely that over the next few years we will see a rise in wellness and medical products featuring these cannabinoids in higher amounts, and aimed at different conditions. Right now, the research is mostly still in the animal and test tube phase, although some preliminary human studies are coming out. But the initial findings so far are very promising for a whole host of issues.

The other key cannabinoids to know about are:

CBG

This is the non-acid form of the mother cannabinoid, CBGA. It is not found in large amounts in many strains, but some high-CBG strains have been bred for extracting the CBG for its medicinal value (by reducing the enzymes that convert CBG into the other cannabinoids). CBG oil is starting to be sold as a health supplement alongside CBD oil in the US, Canada and the UK, although much less is known about it and how to dose it.

CBG has been shown in animal models and in the Petri dish so far to have:

- anti-tumour effects (some types of brain cancers, including glioblastoma in humans, and also breast cancers)
- anti-inflammatory properties
- antibacterial qualities
- antifungal
- pain-relieving
- antidepressant
- effective topically for treating psoriasis

THCA

THCA is the acid precursor to THC but is not intoxicating. It is found in the raw plant and is hard to bottle, but the technology is improving and I have used THCA oil for some of my patients along with CBD- and THC-based medical cannabis. Its medicinal properties include:

- anti-inflammatory
- anticonvulsant

- some anti-tumour effects (*in vitro* studies and animal models)
- anti-obesity[11]

CBDA

CBDA is the acid precursor to CBD found in the raw plant and is also less stable than CBD as far as bottling it goes. So far in animal models it demonstrates medicinal properties, although we know very little about the effects in humans yet. CBDA's medicinal properties include:

- anti-nausea
- anti-inflammatory
- some anti-cancer effects (*in vitro* studies and animal models)

CBN

This is very low in fresh cannabis and is a breakdown product of THC, so the older the cannabis medicine is, the more THC may convert into CBN. It may cause slight intoxication like THC, though less so, but appears so far to be more calming, so can be useful in night-time medical cannabis products for rest and sleep as well as pain. Its properties include:

- sedative
- sleep-promoting
- antibacterial
- analgesic
- anti-inflammatory
- anticonvulsant
- effective topically for psoriasis and burns

CBC

This is a minor cannabinoid that we know less about due to a lack of human studies, but so far the animal research is showing that it is likely to have medicinal value too. It may not work on the cannabinoid receptors directly, just like CBD, but it acts in other ways in the brain and body, which is why putting it together with other cannabinoids may be more effective due to their synergy effect. Properties include:

- anti-cancer effects (*in vitro* studies and animal models)
- anti-inflammatory
- analgesic on its own, and may enhance THC pain-relieving effects when combined

THCV

This minor cannabinoid has been zeroed in on by a few drug companies due to its anti-obesity effect (aka weight loss) in animals, and possibly in humans, although the research is in a very early stage. It is non-intoxicating, and also appears to have other effects in animals that could impact brain-ageing diseases such as dementia. Some of its medicinal properties include:

- a positive effect on bone growth
- may play a role in reducing plaques in Alzheimer's disease
- appetite suppressant
- anti-obesity
- anti-inflammation
- analgesic

CBDV

CBDV is made by some varieties of cannabis and is also non-intoxicating. It seems most promising so far in animal and Petri dish human tissue studies for potentially helping in inflammatory bowel disease by taming gut inflammation. Some of its medicinal properties include:

- anticonvulsant
- anti-nausea
- may reduce intestinal (gut) inflammation[12]

For additional information, see references[13, 14, 15, 16].

A tale of the terpenes

Have you ever wondered why a fresh orange smells so darn good, or why your best friend is obsessed with French lavender? The wonderful (and sometimes quite pungent) aromas of plants are from a group of plant chemicals we call terpenes. They are the essential oils of all plants, including cannabis, and are also found in trees, fruits, flowers, etc. The cannabis plant contains at least 140 (and probably closer to 200) terpenes, in many different combinations depending on the strain, creating scents that can range from pungent and earthy to super-citrusy and fresh. However, terpenes are not just 'scent candy' for humans; they help protect the plant from insects and also attract pollinators. The type of terpenes you get in a certain strain of cannabis depends on the genes of that strain, and also the growing conditions, such as the soil and the weather (if it's grown outdoors), because the plant chemicals adapt to different environments as a way of surviving and thriving.

> **FOREST BATHING**
>
> In Japan, 'forest bathing' in pine forests has become popular for its anti-stress effects and to lift the mood. The dominant terpene in pine trees is called alpha-pinene, which is known to have anti-depressant properties. Cannabis strains high in alpha-pinene are recommended for lifting low moods as well as for helping with memory!

Terpenes are made in the trichomes (resin glands) we learned about earlier, alongside the cannabinoids. Just as with cannabinoids, the unfertilised female flowers have the highest concentration of terpenes, which is why cannabis flowers have a stronger smell than the leaves.

Even though I've never been a recreational cannabis smoker, I love the aroma of the cannabis plant. It's one of my favourite plant scents, and in Canada, where it's legal, I sometimes use it as an incense for meditation – in a well-ventilated room. It's been used this way for religious/spiritual ceremonies for thousands of years by many cultures, including in ancient Babylon.

Although terpenes are present in relatively small amounts in CBD products, they seem to have a possible effect on our brains and bodies even at these very low concentrations. Terpenes that are at levels of only 0.05% are considered potentially significant.[17, 18] In animal studies, terpenes changed behaviour significantly even when the blood terpene levels were very low to barely detectable.[19] Because terpenes are fat-soluble, they can cross the blood–brain barrier and affect the brain directly, especially when we inhale them with a vaporiser (e.g. using medical cannabis or CBD flower), or when we use a special way of absorbing cannabinoids like through a 'transdermal' patch applied to the skin which allows it to absorb into the bloodstream, not just the skin area where it was stuck on to. Eating or ingesting CBD or cannabis medicine products with terpenes (e.g. when using a CBD full-spectrum oil or cannabis oil) also appears to possibly act in the gut on multiple pathways involved in inflammation and pain perception. However, the research in humans is still scant for now on how exactly it works. Terpenes from other plants, such as ginkgo, are taken by mouth and are thought to be biologically active in the brain as well. Certain types of terpenes (the monoterpenes) may also make THC cross the blood–brain barrier and act on the brain more effectively.

Like cannabinoids, terpenes are lipophilic (fat-loving), so again that's why cannabis medicines and CBD oils are best taken with a fat-containing meal, which may help it absorb better, at least in theory. Buying a product with a high-tech formulation to enhance the absorbability may reduce the dose you need to get an effect, though keep in mind that every person's reaction will be slightly different!

In addition to creating the smell of cannabis, the unique combination of the main terpenes plus the CBD:THC ratio come together to help create the different strain-specific effects of cannabis.

The process of making full-spectrum CBD and medical cannabis oils using the most common method, known as CO_2 extraction, can damage the terpenes (unless very specialised equipment is used) to varying degrees, and it is hard to test for the exact amount that is present in the final product, but some may still remain, or even get added, unless the product is labelled as a 'CBD isolate'.

In my opinion, CBD wellness products are probably most effective when they are full-spectrum (where no THC is allowed, CBD broad-spectrum is best, which removes the THC but tries to retain the other cannabinoids), including the terpenes and other minor cannabinoids, rather than in the form of CBD isolate products, which in my experience are often less effective and therefore seem to need far higher doses. CBD isolate is much cheaper compared with full- or broad-spectrum CBD, which is a major reason why it is often used in wellness products and sneakily labelled 'pure' so it sounds better to consumers.[20, 21, 22]

Let's take a tour of the most common and interesting terpenes for wellness and medicinal purposes. This is not by any means a complete list, but I've covered the ones we know the most about so far in terms of their wellness superpowers.

Myrcene

Myrcene is one of the most common terpenes in the cannabis plant.

The first high-CBD strains of medical cannabis, used to make full-spectrum CBD oil, were high in myrcene, which is believed to have given those strains a calming, sedating effect. CBD alone is not necessarily sedating (although many people with anxiety find it calming), but combined with myrcene it can feel very relaxing – almost too calming for daytime use! I have had patients using medical cannabis and clients using CBD wellness products who have commented that their oil at higher doses made them feel sleepy, and lo and behold, it turned out they were using a myrcene-rich product.

Boiling point for vaporising: 168°C (334°F)[†]

Aromas: hoppy, musky, cloves, herbal, citrus

Effects: sedating, relaxing, may enhance THC's effects

Also found in: hops, eucalyptus, mango, thyme, citrus, lemongrass, bay leaves

Medicinal effects: antiseptic, analgesic, hepatoprotective (prevents damage to the liver), antibacterial, antifungal, anti-inflammatory, may be a gastro-protectant (against stomach ulcers)[‡ 23]

Beta-caryophyllene

This is one of my favourite terpenes for use with symptoms that have an inflammatory component, such as arthritis, and also for headaches. Thai basil, or holy basil, is also high in this terpene – another of my favourite herbals for well-being and fighting inflammation and stress.

Boiling point for vaporising: 160°C (320°F)

Aromas: peppery, spicy, woody

Effects: may work together with THC to protect the stomach lining and with CBD to enhance anti-inflammatory effects

Also found in: pepper, cinnamon, cloves, hops, basil, oregano

Medicinal effects: anti-inflammatory, analgesic, antibacterial, antifungal, anti-tumour, kidney protectant (nephroprotectant)

Linalool

This terpene is also what gives lavender its amazing aroma. It is used as an ingredient in products for topical pain relief.

Boiling point for vaporising: 198°C (388°F)

Aromas: floral, citrus, spice

Effects: sedating, calming, mood-balancing

---

† This is the temperature at which the terpene vaporises off the flower. If you are using a vaporiser with either a CBD flower or a medical cannabis flower with THC content >0.2%/0.3%, below that temperature you may not get the effects of the terpene. Beyond that temperature, or after heating multiple times, the terpene will have mostly evaporated or been inhaled on subsequent vapour inhalations. See Chapter Five for more details on vaporising.

‡ For all terpenes, the medicinal effects listed are mainly in animals in terms of published research.

Also found in: lavender, citrus, laurel, birch, rosewood

Medicinal effects: local anaesthetic properties (good for topicals as a pain salve), sleep aid, antidepressant, anti-anxiety, immune-regulating properties, analgesic, anticonvulsant, anti-acne

Pinene

Pinene is a really promising terpene that crosses the blood–brain barrier easily to directly impact the nervous system. In addition to its anti-inflammatory and antimicrobial action, like many other terpenes it has a unique skill of potentially blocking the short-term memory impairment from THC. Intriguingly, THC and pinene together show potential as a treatment for dementia and Alzheimer's.

Boiling point for vaporising: 155°C (311°F)

Aromas: sharp, sweet, pine

Effects: enhances memory retention and alertness

Also found in: pine needles, conifer trees, sage

Medicinal effects: anti-inflammatory, antibiotic, antiviral, anti-tumour, buffers THC short-term memory effects, asthma (bronchodilator)

Humulene

Humulene suppresses appetite, whereas many high-THC strains can tend to stimulate it. Strains higher in humulene may help prevent the 'munchies', or appetite increases from THC, when these strains are used in the medical cannabis treatment of severe pain conditions, for example.

Boiling point for vaporising: 198°C (388°F)

Aromas: woody, earthy

Effects: suppresses appetite

Also found in: hops, coriander

Medicinal effects: anti-inflammatory, antibacterial, pain relief

D-Limonene

D-limonene is known to be a mood elevator, so choosing strains higher in this are good for depression and low moods.

Boiling point for vaporising: 176°C (349°F)

Aromas: citrus, lemon, orange
Effects: elevates mood, stress relief
Also found in: citrus rinds, juniper, peppermint
Medicinal effects: antidepressant, anti-anxiety, relief of gastric reflux, antifungal

Flavonoids

Flavonoids are the plant chemicals that give cannabis and other plants their colour, but they also have medicinal properties in humans, mirroring what they do for the plants: protecting against UV light and diseases. For example, quercetin is a yellow flavonoid that is one of the most abundant flavonoids found in cannabis, as well as in tomatoes, red wine and berries. It has been shown to have anti-cancer, antioxidant and antiviral properties *in vitro* and in animal models. There are other flavonoids that are unique to the cannabis plant, such as cannflavin A, which is a potent anti-inflammatory.

The entourage effect: herbal medicine synergy at its finest

The entourage effect is a well-established concept in botanical medicine. When plant chemicals are combined (as they naturally occur in the plant), the chemicals work together to produce a therapeutic effect that is greater than the sum of its parts. This was one of the first things I learned when I studied how to combine herbal medicines for more potent effects (long before I was prescribing cannabis and CBD). It's not just in cannabis that we see this effect, but in all plant medicines. This is the way traditional Chinese medicine (TCM) herbs work too, and why it's hard to turn them into single-ingredient drugs, which has been tried time and time again in China without success. Cannabis, however, as a single plant, is a total powerhouse and really does stand out even from other herbal medicines.

For example, CBD on its own is a good natural anti-seizure chemical, and is the main ingredient of the pharmaceutical drug

Epidiolex, licensed for treating some forms of childhood epilepsy. Approximately half the kids who are given Epidiolex have around a 50% reduction in their seizures. However, some children stop responding to it, or it just doesn't work very well for them. Yet when they are given a high-CBD full-extract cannabis oil with small amounts of THC and THCA, their response improves again – the combination works better than the CBD on its own in some of these cases clinically.

I also see this in many of my patients who are referred to me after failing to respond to one of the man-made THC drugs (e.g. nabilone, dronabinol), or who are experiencing lots of side effects from them. When we start using a full-spectrum cannabis oil that still contains THC (by prescription), their symptoms almost universally improve once we find the right strain or product, and they usually do not have significant, if any, side effects. They are often reluctant to try *any* cannabis medicine product again after their negative THC pill experience, but I explain to them that when you isolate the most potentially intoxicating chemical from the plant and stick it in a pill with no other plant chemicals to buffer and work with it, it can create an increased incidence of side effects, as well as just not working as well for the symptoms (usually chronic pain or nausea from cancer treatments) for which it was intended.

Cannabis roots: a new frontier

Although the roots of the cannabis plant have no cannabinoids (i.e. you can't use the roots to get CBD or THC), they have many secrets of their own. They have traditionally been used in the treatment of gout. Recent research has discovered that these roots are rich in many non-intoxicating but potentially useful substances:[24] terpenoids, sterols and other anti-inflammatory chemicals. Researching uses for these roots may be the next big thing!

For additional information, see references[25, 26, 27, 28].

The sativa vs indica classification

Although it is technically inaccurate and drives scientists crazy, many of the medical cannabis industry products as well as legal cannabis dispensary products in the US and Canada use the sativa vs indica labelling system. CBD wellness products made from hemp that you can buy without a prescription will generally not use this system, though you will see the terms occasionally.

The system is meant to help you know whether the product will be relaxing/sedating or uplifting/energising, since different strains of cannabis can do different things.

If this is the only guide you have to go on, in theory anything labelled as 'indica dominant' may be better for chilling out, calming down, evening time and sleep time. A 'sativa dominant' product, on the other hand, may be best for the morning and daytime, for lifting the mood and even slightly boosting energy and motivation.

In reality, pure sativa and pure indica products don't really exist any longer, since after many years of interbreeding, modern cannabis strains are mostly hybrids. Sort of like a third-generation Cockapoo.

Originally you could tell a sativa from an indica by the way the plant looked. Classical sativa varieties (the uplifting strains) had narrow leaves and were tall, skinny plants. Originally they tended to grow well naturally in tropical Asia, countries such as Thailand and Vietnam.

Classical indica varieties (the calming/sedating strains) were short, squat plants with broad leaves. These were originally found in regions of Afghanistan and Pakistan and used for making hashish. Their size and shape made it easier to harvest the sticky resin on the flowers to make hashish oil.

So here's the issue: due to all the genetic interbreeding and strain mixing, generally speaking you can no longer look at a plant's leaves, height or appearance and predict the type of effect it will have on you. However, many patients still choose products from a dispensary using this method (since it is often the only way they are labelled) and report that it still works better than no system at all.

RUSSIAN CANNABIS

Some cannabis scientists insist there should be a third cannabis subtype alongside sativa and indica: ruderalis. Others argue that ruderalis is actually a subtype of the *Cannabis sativa ssp. sativa* variety and doesn't need its own class. Ruderalis was discovered in southern Siberia in 1924. It contains very little THC and is higher in CBD and the cannabinoid CBN, which also seems to have medicinal value for pain and sleep. The ruderalis variety does something unique – it autoflowers, which means it starts to make flowers even if it is not exposed to the minimum 12 hours of darkness each day that other types of cannabis need to trigger them from the dormant (vegetative) phase to the flowering phase.

The chemovar classification method

A more scientific way to predict what effects a strain may have is by looking at its actual chemical make-up. This is known to scientists as its chemovar, a classification based on the most abundant chemicals that particular plant and strain contains. You can think of a chemovar as being like a plant's fingerprint, each one different and unique. Even if you start with the same seeds (or clones) from one strain but you grow them under different conditions, the final plant fingerprints will vary slightly. So even though the plant genes are the same, the nurture part is different, and that contributes to the final chemovar. If you want to grow plants that contain the same chemovar, you need to start with the same strain *and* grow them under the same conditions.

It's rather like taking identical twins and separating them at birth, then raising them completely differently. They are likely to develop different personalities and may even start to look different too. It's not just the genes you started with that matter. That is why even if you buy a strain of cannabis with the same name as one you've tried before, but from a different grower or batch, the effects on you may be slightly different. This is especially an issue with recreational cannabis, home-grown cannabis and black market cannabis, because often you don't know the plant's fingerprint completely. Even with medical cannabis, it can be a challange. Cannabis typing and categorisation is moving towards the chemovar classification to help standardise the medicinal strains and final products, so that they are close to the same for each batch and more predictable in their effects on us.

Thousands of slightly different versions of these chemovars[§] have emerged over the years, due to humans growing plants in different conditions and breeding them for certain traits – just like you have dozens of types of tomatoes with slightly different colours, flavours and phytochemical profiles.

Type I–III chemovars

Within the chemovar classification system, plant scientists and medical researchers sort *Cannabis sativa* into three groups: type I, II and III. This is based on a plant's THC:CBD ratio, without taking into account the other plant chemicals, terpene profiles or other minor cannabinoids. That's why there are only three groups rather than hundreds, since the system only factors in the two main cannabinoids. This arrangement is favoured by medical doctors because it lets them know how psychotomimetic (capable of producing an intoxicating effect) a particular strain may be. The more THC and the less CBD, the higher the potential for intoxication. The system is as follows:

- Type I: THC-dominant strains of the plant (very little CBD)
- Type II: strains that produce equal or close to equal amounts of CBD and THC
- Type III: CBD-dominant strains (very little THC)

---

§ Chemovars are sometimes also called cultivars, because they are a product of cultivating (breeding and growing) the plant for specific traits. However, for the rest of this book, I will tend to refer to them as 'strains' to keep things simple.

Chemovar classifications based on terpenes

An even more recently proposed way to classify strains is by their terpene profile (see p.34). Some researchers have made a case for categorising strains based on three main terpene groups: limonene, myrcene and terpinolene,[29] while others have proposed using alpha-pinene, beta-caryophyllene and limonene.

Classification systems bottom line: the trend in categorising cannabis strains and types is moving away from 'sativa vs indica' and towards the main plant chemicals from both a CBD and THC and a terpene perspective. This categorisation gives people a better idea of the actual effects of a particular strain and is a more scientifically accurate way of classifying cannabis.

Industrial hemp for CBD and other cannabinoids

Industrial hemp strains are mostly male plants (no flowers) or a mix of male and female. They do not produce much THC – to count as hemp, a plant must contain less than 0.2% THC (UK) or less than 0.3% THC (USA) – but do make small amounts of CBD in the leaves as well as any flowers if female plants are included. What that means in terms of the medicinal cannabinoids is that you need to harvest way more plants to get the same amount of CBD and other non-THC minor cannabinoids. Most hemp varieties contain only about 3.5% CBD. By comparison, female flowers from medical cannabis strains that are cultivated to be high-CBD varieties can have upwards of 15–20% CBD. This is a challenge to be overcome, since it's not good for the planet or the medicine if it takes 100 plants to do the job that 10 could do! Luckily, plant scientists are solving this issue by cultivating new higher-CBD varieties that contain up to 10% CBD but only 0.2 or 0.3% THC so that they still qualify as hemp.

In many countries, it is currently only legal to grow low-THC hemp varieties, so most of the CBD products you see on the shelves in the UK and the US, available without a medical prescription, come from these varieties. If, on the other hand, you get a high-CBD medical cannabis oil on prescription (in Canada and some US states, these are also now available over the counter), this is normally made from the female unfertilised flowers and will have slightly more THC (around 0.5 or 1%) than a hemp CBD oil, although it is unlikely to be enough to get you high for most people (but there are exceptions and some people who are ultrasensitive may notice a perceptible effect). However, due to advancements in plant genetics and cultivation, this distinction is getting murkier. New strains are being invented to produce larger amounts of CBD while still falling below the THC levels that classify them as hemp.

Scientists are still arguing about the exact differences genetically between hemp strains and cannabis strains with over 0.3% THC. There are lots of overlapping genes between the two types, although hemp varieties seem to come from a slightly wider gene pool compared to the high-THC strains bred for the recreational market over the past few decades.[30]

Whatever the source of CBD used to make full-spectrum oil, it is important that the method of extraction doesn't produce harmful chemicals. For this reason, CO_2 supercritical extraction, which uses pressurised carbon dioxide, is considered one of the best methods, rather than using solvents like butane and hexane that can leave behind toxic residues – as has been demonstrated in multiple lab tests and studies investigating common CBD products. If the source of CBD is high-CBD female flowers, a simple alcohol or oil extraction method is also possible, and is safer than other solvents. New and better ways of extraction are being developed all the time, and it won't be long before CO_2 extraction may not be the easy winner for large-scale extraction.

Industrial hemp is also cultivated for non-medical and non-wellness uses, to make clothes, paper, textiles, rope, hemp plastic, hemp batteries and biofuel, while the seeds are sold as a health food.

CHERNOBYL CLEAN-UP WITH HEMP

After the nuclear disaster at Chernobyl, hemp was planted to bioremediate, or clean, the soil. This is because hemp is a bioaccumulant – a plant that soaks up toxins from the soil and accumulates them within itself. It is used worldwide to clean soil that is contaminated with heavy metals and other toxins. That is why it is so important to know where your CBD oil comes from, and to check that it's been tested for contaminants, since hemp grown in toxic soil is not fit for human consumption. All hemp full-spectrum and broad-spectrum CBD oil should be tested by an independent lab to ensure there are no toxic residues left in the final product.

CHAPTER FOUR

CANNABIS AND YOUR BODY

Now that you understand the plant, it's time to explore how our bodies respond to cannabis in all its forms.

Scientists have discovered that we have our very own cannabis-like system naturally in our body, called the endocannabinoid system, or the ECS for short.

Our ECS helps control some of the most important physical, mental and emotional functions in the brain and body, everything from body movement, pain control and immune system function to mental health, sleep, gut function and even brain protection. You literally cannot overstate how important our ECS is, and it does all these crucial things by controlling something called homeostasis, or our overall brain and body balance.

Despite the ECS being a mystery to many, it's a critically important system, as important as the endocrine system (our hormone system), the endorphin system (which makes our 'feel-good chemicals') and all the other major body systems we rely on to function normally. The endocannabinoid system may end up being one of the most important systems for maintaining health and wellness and avoiding major disease.

Endo means 'inside us', and cannabinoids are chemicals similar to CBD and THC from the cannabis plant, thus these endocannabinoids are chemicals that our own bodies make naturally (cannabinoids like THC and CBD from plants are known as phytocannabinoids, which we learned about in Chapter Three).

The main roles of the ECS can be remembered by the mnemonic Eat, Sleep, Relax, Protect, Forget.

Eat: It influences our appetite, how we metabolise our food, insulin regulation and many other food-related metabolic functions.

Sleep: It influences our sleep/wake cycles and affects different stages of sleep.

Relax: It affects our nervous system's ability to wind down and return to a calm baseline, and helps balance our calming brain chemicals, such as GABA (gamma aminobutyric acid). This protects us from hyperarousal and anxiety and helps our nervous system to self-soothe so we can manage chronic stress without it turning toxic.

Protect: It regulates our immune system against outside invaders (e.g. infections from bacteria and viruses) and inside threats (cancer, autoimmune issues), and protects our brain against toxins and inflammation, helping to regulate healthy programmed cell death.

Forget: It helps the brain and body process traumatic events and fear memory to aid in trauma healing and stress recovery so we don't get stuck in fight-or-flight mode. This often goes wrong in PTSD, which is why medical cannabis can be so helpful to sufferers.

The ECS is all about helping maintain equilibrium or balance on every level in your brain and body. It even has a major role in female reproductive health and bone health.

Most importantly, just like any other body system, we don't really notice our endocannabinoid system until something isn't working right. It's like breathing, something we do in the background but only become aware of if we try to hold our breath.

Most of the time, it's just there, doing its balancing act without any applause. However, there are many diseases and symptoms that, according to recent research, may be related to or at least involve a dysfunctional endocannabinoid system – problems like chronic pain, fibromyalgia, anxiety and depression, neurodegenerative diseases like multiple sclerosis and Alzheimer's, epilepsy, chronic headaches, irritable bowel, inflammation, autoimmune diseases and many more.

When the ECS isn't functioning properly, adding in cannabinoids from the cannabis plant like CBD, THC and the hundreds of other minor cannabinoids and terpenes in a cannabis oil, cannabis flower or other method of getting into into the body may help restore balance and alleviate symptoms without major side effects. In short, the cannabis plant may help your ECS put things back together when something gets out of balance.

So even if you have never heard of CBD oil and never smoked cannabis in your life, your body still depends on its very own endocannabinoids to function normally and stay healthy, happy and balanced.

The endocannabinoid system was only discovered in the last 30 years, which explains why the research is still quite young compared to our knowledge of other body systems. Most doctors still don't really know anything about it, and I didn't learn about it in medical school; they just sort of left it out back then, and many top medical schools still do!

Humans are not the only species with an endocannabinoid system. All other animals, even fish, have it too, and it's just as important for them as it is for humans. This explains why I can give my Cavapoo puppy CBD to help with separation anxiety and it works like a charm, just as it does on humans with anxiety. This natural system we have that recognises cannabinoids is why plant cannabinoids from cannabis are so effective for many issues in our bodies and brains. It is like we were designed to use plants as medicines, and that is reflected by the fact that over half of all modern drugs come from plants.[1]

The discovery of the endocannabinoid system: unveiling the 'hidden world'

So let's backtrack in time a bit, to 1964, when the hippie movement was in full force and, over in Israel, a curious scientist by the name of Raphael Mechoulam wanted to answer a simple question: 'What is it in the cannabis plant that makes you high?' He found out – and called the plant chemical tetrahydrocannabinol, or THC.

So now we knew that THC was what caused the 'high' feeling, but the bigger question was how exactly did THC and the rest of the plant cannabinoids actually work in our brain and body. This remained a mystery until the late 1980s. The long search was over with the discovery of the first cannabinoid receptor in the human body, named the CB1 receptor.

The CB1 receptor is actually a protein our body makes that acts like a docking station for plant THC to lock onto. This allows plant THC to 'talk' to brain and body and interact with our very own ECS!

So the discovery of this CB1 receptor was cold, hard scientific proof that we had our very own endocannabinoid system, made up of three main parts:

1. Receptors. These are the docking stations, and the two receptors we know most about are CB1 and CB2 (a third type provisionally named CB3 is currently being explored).
2. Endocannabinoids. Natural cannabis-like chemicals we produce in our very own bodies that talk to the receptors. The two main ones are called 2-AG and anandamide.
3. Enzymes. We have two types of enzymes in our body that interact with our endocannabinoids. The first type makes the endocannabinoid chemicals in our body from building blocks; the second type breaks down the endocannabinoids and gets rid of them once they've done their job.

So up until the 1990s, this whole endocannabinoid system was like a hidden world that we relied on for the most basic of daily life functions without even knowing it. Since the CB1 receptor discovery, we have found the CB2 and the possible CB3 receptor, and there are probably many more we don't know about yet that are hiding in our brains and bodies just waiting to make their grand entrance!

So the deal is, regardless of whether it's external cannabinoids from the plant (phytocannabinoids) or internal cannabinoids made inside our own body (endocannabinoids), they go and hang out in the cannabinoid CB receptors (docking stations) throughout our brain and body.

There are CB receptors in our brain, nervous system, major organs, connective tissues, glands, gut, immune cells and even our bone marrow. They do different jobs in each place, but keeping the balance (homeostasis) is their overall mission, no matter where they act or how they do it. That's their duty: maintaining balance, keeping the peace and being the mastermind of a smoothly operating brain and body under the stresses of life. If they had a slogan, it would be 'Keep Calm and Carry On'.

Cannabinoids work to help balance the flow of neurotransmitters (brain chemicals like serotonin and dopamine), hormones and immune cells. It's a big job and a complex one and we still don't fully understand exactly how it works. But what we do know is that when the ECS is not functioning normally – if the system gets out of whack and doesn't make enough cannabinoids or in the right spot, or the CB1 and CB2 receptor balance is off – it can contribute to a whole host of seemingly unconnected issues, because the overall flow and balance of our nervous system and immune system has been disturbed and *boom*, it's a chaotic free-for-all.

This chaos can show up in many different ways: depression and anxiety, sleep problems, chronic pain, immune dysregulation, gut issues, appetite changes and even neurological disorders and brain inflammation ... the list goes on. That's because the ECS sits like a skin overlaying many other messaging and chemical systems in the brain and body to help regulate these systems too.

We do know that the endocannabinoids play a huge role in pain signalling, and that in conditions like fibromyalgia, the baseline tone of background pain signalling is too high. I've found cannabis and CBD to be the most effective single tool in helping treat fibromyalgia symptoms in my own patients, when dozens of drugs, supplements, psychological treatments and lifestyle changes have all failed to make much of a difference.

Meet our very own endocannabinoids: 2-AG and anandamide

The full names for the dynamic duo of endocannabinoids we make in our own bodies, and that we know the most about so far, are 2-arachidonoylglycerol (2-AG) and anandamide. Anandamide comes from the Sanskrit word *ananda*, which means 'internal bliss'.[2] It's a great name because that is its job: to create balance and happiness within your nervous system.

Once they've done their job, 2-AG and anandamide are broken down by special enzymes and a fresh batch is made inside our cells. Anandamide is broken down by an enzyme called fatty acid amide hydrolase (FAAH), and 2-AG is broken down by three enzymes: mono-acylglycerol lipase (MGL) and alpha/beta hydrolase domain (ABHD) 6 and 12.[3] Don't stress about these details; the most important thing to remember is that our cannabis-like chemicals get made and then broken down by our own body without any outside help. This is similar to the way our body is able to make other key hormones like oestrogen and testosterone, and brain chemicals like serotonin.

Endocannabinoids and plant phytocannabinoids like CBD and THC work in the brain through a special type of code called retrograde signalling. Cannabinoids prevent overexcited signalling on something called the presynaptic neuron. This means they basically stop brain cells from releasing too much of a particular brain chemical at once (like flooding the brain too fast with serotonin or dopamine, or GABA).

You can think of endocannabinoids as the dimmer switch for the nervous system and immune system. They are sort of like the party police, rocking up to a house party when a thousand people have turned up and things are getting too rowdy. They keep the numbers in check, always a good thing when it is your house (your brain, body and nervous system). No one wants a thousand people showing up at their house all at once! But this special police force also makes sure there are enough people at the party so it is not a dud, letting just enough guests in to fill up the dance floor.

When the party police or dimmer switch doesn't function properly, you get something called excitotoxicity – excessive stimulation or excitement of brain chemical messaging, which we see in epilepsy and neurological disorders. This prevention of overexcitement is one way in which plant cannabinoids reduce the symptoms of these diseases. In many other situations where our own endocannabinoids are struggling to keep the balance by themselves, such as chronic stress, anxiety, PTSD and autoimmune diseases, outside helpers like plant cannabinoids (THC and CBD) may help give them a boost.

This is the nerdy, nitty-gritty detail of how the endocannabinoid system helps us maintain homeostasis, or our inner balance.

CB1 receptors

CB1 receptors are found mainly in the brain and central nervous system. More specifically, you find them in large amounts in brain areas that deal with emotional memory, fear, pain, pleasure, mood, physical balance and basic human drives (like for food and sex). These brain areas have names such as the basal ganglia, amygdala and limbic system, the hippocampus and the cerebellum, just to name a few.

Anandamide, which we make ourselves, and THC, from the cannabis plant, both bind or dock into CB1 receptors really well – they fit like a glove. When anandamide or THC hang out in the CB1 receptor, they have multiple effects on the brain's other chemicals too (such as the happy hormone serotonin). CB1 receptor activation from THC or anandamide can boost your mood, decrease anxiety and stress responses, relieve pain, activate brain pleasure centres and increase appetite.

CB1 receptor activation is also involved in a whole host of other higher brain functions such as learning, memory and balance, and even helps protect brain cells from toxins and inflammation.[4]

When you inhale or consume cannabis that contains high levels of THC, especially without much CBD to mitigate its effects, the THC binds to the CB1 receptors, producing intoxication. This intoxication effect from a drug or plant chemical is known to scientists as a psychotomimetic effect (aka feeling high or having a temporarily altered perception of things). To reduce or even, in many cases, eliminate the intoxication or altered feeling, which for some people can be unpleasant, you can add CBD, which tends to help buffer this effect.

CBD is what is called a negative allosteric modulator (NAM), which in English means that it has the ability to decrease the intoxication effect of THC. It appears that it does this by decreasing the responsiveness to THC at the CB1 receptor. This is the nerdy scientific reason for why and how CBD can buffer THC intoxication effects. So even if you take the same amount of THC but you add CBD, you may not feel high as you likely would if you took the THC by itself. Based on our current knowledge, this NAM effect is another reason why CBD seems to have a balancing effect on our endocannabinoids – it may help to regulate the CB1 receptors in general throughout the nervous system.[5, 6]

This is why the medical cannabis strains I use most in my practice tend to have a significant amount of CBD. Recreational cannabis strains are high in THC without much or any CBD, since they are bred for the main goal of making people feel intoxicated. However, the lack of CBD in these black market and recreational strains can cause some people to feel negative or dysphoric. That is not what you want, especially if keeping a positive mood balance is an issue or you have suffered from depression or anxiety in the past.

Another trick for reducing THC's intoxication effects, dating back to tenth-century Persia, is to drink lemon[7] or lime juice after taking THC. A plant chemical called D-limonene, found in citrus fruit (and also in some strains of cannabis), may affect how THC works at the receptor, although no hard research studies on this have been done recently (not sure who would fund that!). Adding CBD can also greatly reduce or even eliminate the short-term memory impairment that high THC on its own can create (aka 'stoner brain').[8] However, THC is not intrinsically bad. In fact, in small doses, especially when combined with CBD, it can play a hugely therapeutic role in reducing insomnia, anxiety, PTSD symptoms, period pain and chronic pain of many types, and even in some cases boosting mood in depression (see Chapter Ten). THC has many other superpowers when it's used correctly, especially if your own anandamide isn't doing its job properly at those CB1 receptors and your system needs a bit of a boost. THC's effect on activating the CB1 receptor also appears to be neuroprotective,[9] especially after a head injury, which is totally the opposite of what many people would expect!

THC can also be micro-dosed very effectively in many cases without making you feel high alongside a CBD product, but is only an option in places where THC medical cannabis is legal.

CB2 receptors

CB2 receptors are found throughout the body – in the immune system, gut, bone marrow, reproductive organs, urinary tract and endocrine (hormone) system – as well as in the brain, in the hippocampus (the centre for memory and learning).

They are also found in special brain helper cells called microglia, and in other brain cells, where they help with protection against toxins, inflammation and premature brain cell death.[10,11,12,13] So basically, the CB2 receptors are all over the place and we only understand a small part of everything they do. 2-AG (one of our own naturally produced endocannabinoids, along with anandamide) tends to prefer the CB2 receptor over the CB1, so it generally hangs out here.

THC also binds to CB2 receptors in the immune system in response to injury or inflammation, seeming to work as a natural anti-inflammatory 20 times as powerful as aspirin and twice as powerful as the strong anti-inflammatory steroid hydrocortisone.[14]

CBD, the main non-intoxicating chemical in the cannabis plant, binds only weakly at best to both CB1 and CB2 receptors and has the majority of its effects through other channels.[15] CBD binds to numerous other receptors too, to enhance cell signalling (how cells talk to each other and send messages) and work on voltage-gated ion channels, protein kinase pathways, serotonin receptors and vanilloid receptor pathways, as well as orphan receptors, which are receptors we know exist but haven't yet completely figured out the specific proteins that bind to them.

CBD is a bit like a surly, rebellious teenager that is unenthusiastic about visiting the places its parents want to take it, like school and grandma's house. It visits the CB1 or CB2 receptors a bit but doesn't like to stick around too long. It likes to visit lots of other places and just hang out, and even sneaks out of the house at night to go who knows where! It also decreases the intoxicant effects of THC by having some of the opposite action at the CB1 and CB2 receptors, so it balances out THC and may even enhance its medicinal actions in the brain and body.

CBD acts as a balancer or an orchestral conductor, if you will, of the entire endocannabinoid system, helping to tune the system up or down as needed.[16]

In a nutshell, plant CBD seems to help tweak or modulate the amounts of anandamide and 2-AG floating around in the body and brain.

The complicated balancing/harmonising act that CBD pulls off in our body is actually quite common for a botanical medicine, even though CBD does it better than most. Herbal medicines with plant chemicals can do a gazillion different things at once in the brain and body, yet this superpower is virtually unheard of with man-made pharmaceutical drugs.

This ability to act on widespread areas provides an explanation for why CBD and cannabis medicines seem to work for so many issues, helping symptoms from seizures to inflammation, anxiety and even acne! Doctors who don't do cannabis medicine and canna-sceptics will often say to me, 'I don't believe in cannabis as a medicine; it just sounds like a cure-all snake oil', or 'It's impossible for one thing to work for that many problems; it must be an overhyped miracle cure invented by the stoners.'

But now that we understand the huge variety of areas the endocannabinoid system controls and interacts with, it's quite simple to see how and why cannabis can help with so many completely differ-ent issues and symptoms.

And because our endocannabinoid system is a proven biologi-cal system inside all of us, not believing in cannabinoids is like not believing in science. Luckily, many people – including doctors – are coming around once they have been taught about how it all works and once they understand the science. In fact, most doctors I meet are open, curious and willing to explore cannabis as a treatment option for patients who have been deemed untreatable after trying every drug under the sun. They see it as a ray of hope for those whom drugs have failed.

For additional information see references[17, 18, 19, 20, 21, 22].

When our endocannabinoid system goes wrong . . .

General dysfunction/dysregulation

Everyone's endocannabinoid system is slightly different; you can think of it sort of like your fingerprint – unique to you. We know that many complex chronic symptoms and even full-blown diseases are directly related to a dysfunctional endocannabinoid system. This system can get too high (too much endocannabinoids) or too low (not enough endocannabinoids) when it gets out of balance. Dysregulation of our homeostasis system has been linked to everything from epilepsy to depression and heart disease, including:[23]

- mood disorders such as anxiety and depression
- schizophrenia
- migraine and chronic headache disorders
- seizure disorders
- autism
- cardiovascular disease
- autoimmune diseases: rheumatoid arthritis, Crohn's disease, etc.
- chronic pain, including treatment-resistant pain syndromes such as complex regional pain syndrome
- multiple sclerosis

- Huntington's disease
- Parkinson's disease
- PMS, PMDD (premenstrual dysmorphic disorder) and period symptoms
- chronic nausea
- motion sickness

Endocannabinoid deficiency syndrome

Dr Ethan Russo, an American clinician-researcher and pioneer in cannabis medicine and a practising neurologist, started to investigate and publish groundbreaking research papers about the possibility of an endocannabinoid deficiency syndrome connecting the many common symptoms seen by doctors of neurology and also widely by medics in general practice: irritable bowel syndrome, migraines, fibromyalgia and other 'treatment-resistant' chronic symptoms that seemed to respond almost instantly to medical cannabis when drugs had failed to show much improvement. I have found this theory to be true in my practice, where as an integrative medicine doctor I specialise in these types of conditions and tend to have patients referred to me who have 'tried everything'. The response to medical cannabis has been so life-changing in so many of my patients suffering with these conditions that it still leaves me in awe even after years of working with the cannabis plant. In addition to these specific conditions, I have also found that cannabis has helped my patients who suffer from chronic fatigue syndrome, ME and mitochondrial dysfunction, causing poor exercise tolerance and poor stress tolerance, when again not much else had worked before.

Endocannabinoid overactivity

Multiple studies have looked at the role of too much endocannabinoids in promoting obesity and even type 2 diabetes through their effect on metabolism, satiety and hunger signals. The hungrier we are, the more we are driven to eat, and the extra weight gain and adipose (fat) tissue may trigger more cannabinoids to be made in a repeating cycle, leading to more weight gain and less control over food intake. In addition to being driven to eat more, a too-high endocannabinoid system also seems to impact how the body can process sugars and fat, which may lead us down a path to higher blood sugar and type 2 diabetes. Differences in gut bacteria (the microbiome) may also play a role in changing endocannabinoid levels[24] and affecting metabolism, and we don't yet have all the answers. [25, 26, 27]

Natural ways of increasing our own endocannabinoid system

In addition to adding plant cannabinoids like CBD and THC from the cannabis plant, there are other ways to boost or support our natural endocannabinoid levels.

Aerobic exercise

Our natural anandamide levels are increased by aerobic exercise, and along with endorphins, they may be partly responsible for the runner's high. It's a good excuse for a dance party.

Cacao and maca

Cacao, which is used to make chocolate and as a health supplement ingredient, and maca root, a popular health supplement and health food ingredient, also affect our endocannabinoid system.

Hence why you may crave chocolate when you are stressed, or why smoothies containing maca powder may make some people feel friskier and increase libido – because another thing our endocannabinoid system takes care of is our libido. Cacao and maca both work on our endocannabinoid system by blocking the enzyme called FAAH that breaks down our natural anandamide, so it sticks around for longer. In plain English, this means that taking cacao or maca will result in more natural cannabis-like chemicals floating around in our brain and body.[28]

Other herbs

Several other herbs may also influence our endocannabinoid system, such as chemicals called alkylamides in the echinacea plant and actual cannabinoids in liverwort, another medicinal plant. Kava, a plant root used for hundreds of years in South Asian cultures for anxiety and sleep, also interacts with our endocannabinoid system.

Carrots

The humble carrot contains a chemical that acts as what scientists call an inverse agonist at the CB1 receptor, which in English means it does the opposite of what THC does. Does that mean a carrot binge could help reduce THC intoxication? Probably not, unless you ate a couple of thousand! But the chemistry is there in the plant. Our overall diet may contribute significantly to how our endocannabinoid system works, which is a new frontier in nutritional medicine.

High omega-3, lower omega-6 diet

There is some preliminary evidence in animals that a diet higher in omega-3 and lower in omega-6 may improve the function of the overall endocannabinoid system, reduce inflammation and help CB1 vs CB2 receptor activation balance. Foods rich in omega-3 fatty acids include fatty fish (the best source). Vegan sources of omega-3 are less effective but include hemp hearts (from the cannabis plant, no less), flax seeds, chia seeds, walnuts and avocados, blackcurrant seed oil and borage seed oil, which you can take as a supplement.

Western diets tend towards overconsumption of omega-6 fatty acids from common foods such as mixed vegetable oil, eggs, meat, snack foods and most 'diet' foods. The optimal ratio of omega-3 to omega-6 fatty acids in humans is probably around 1:1, but most modern diets are more like 1:20.[29] I recommend eating small wild (not farmed) fatty fish, as well as supplementing with krill or purified omega-3 oil from fish.

MAN-MADE CANNABINOIDS

In addition to our own cannabinoids and plant cannabinoids, there's a third type that can bind to our cannabinoid receptors, but they don't come from nature; they are man-made or synthetic cannabinoids. The most well-known synthetic cannabinoids are the drugs nabilone and dronabinol.

However, these drugs only contain THC but lack the other hundreds of plant compounds found in whole herbal cannabis extracts. This is probably why they rarely seem to work as well, and with as few side effects, as the whole-extract cannabis medicine products made from a well-chosen strain to match person and symptoms. There have been no large head-to-head comparisons, but this is the information that comes back again and again from patients who have tried both, and has also been my clinical experience.

Another type of synthetic cannabinoid is an illegal drug known as 'spice'. Unlike natural cannabis, which is very safe, spice can be dangerous and even toxic. It is often added to street cannabis to give people more of a high. That is why black market cannabis from God-knows-where is best avoided (apart from the legal issue!), because you never quite know what is in it.

CHAPTER FIVE

METHODS OF CBD AND CANNABIS DELIVERY

There are so many forms of CBD and medical cannabis out there that it's often overwhelming and difficult to know where to start. Many of my patients and clients are confused about which effective products are available on an over-the-counter basis (in the UK, that's hemp-based CBD wellness products) and which must be prescribed by a doctor (in the UK, that's medical cannabis that contains some THC).

Let's start off by taking a look at CBD.

One of the great things about CBD is that it's generally quite safe for most people, especially at the low doses found in over-the-counter CBD products. When I prescribe high-CBD medical cannabis products to my patients, I still start at small doses, because if it works for someone at a lower dose, it saves them money. I've also used higher doses, well over 100 mg/day, to help with seizure control in epilepsy, for example. CBD is so safe that even in studies where they dosed healthy subjects with 600 mg at a time (way higher than any dose I've ever used), there were no ill effects in healthy adults with anxiety. You could probably swallow an entire bottle of a hemp CBD oil from a health shop and the only side effect would likely be a financial one (of course I don't recommend you do that however)!

Even the usually conservative World Health Organization, the leading authority on what is and isn't medically safe, declared in 2017 that CBD appears to have low toxicity in humans and poses no public health risks.[11] That's a pretty big statement when you think how cannabis has been demonised until recently.

Generally speaking, the more CBD there is in a product, the more expensive it will be, although it also depends on the type of CBD that is used and how absorbable to the body it is, which can also make a huge difference in how well it works. For example, a high-tech transdermal patch or inhaled CBD flower products are both highly absorbable forms of CBD, so less is needed to get the same effect compared to an oil you ingest, which gets broken down in the stomach and liver first and only a small fraction gets absorbed (therefore requiring you to take more for the same effect). A full- or broad-spectrum CBD product is made from an extract that also still contains other minor cannabinoids and terpenes from the plant to create the herbal synergy we learned about in Chapter Three.

There are also products made from CBD isolate, meaning they contain CBD and nothing else, which is thought to be less effective. CBD isolate is a much cheaper ingredient, though I have seen multiple CBD products on the shelves that have sneakily used CBD isolate while charging crazy prices. Even if the packaging declares that the product is made from 'pure CBD', always check the small print to see if they have actually used CBD isolate rather than full- or broad-spectrum. Another clue that the product may be using an isolate is if it claims to contain a huge amount (i.e. over 1000 mg) of CBD but is much cheaper than the leading reputable brands. I have seen products advertised online that contain 3000–6000 mg per small (10–30 ml) bottle for under £50. I have also seen 'hemp oil' that turns out on closer inspection to be hemp seed oil, not CBD, advertised with misleading information at very low prices. As consumers become savvier, this is likely to become harder to get away with, but it is still something to watch out for. CBD isolate is not 'unsafe' but may just not be as effective as a full- or broad--spectrum product, based on anecdotal evidence and my experience.

¶ Although CBD hemp products are in general very safe, please see Chapter Six for a full list of cautions, side effects and contraindications before embarking on your cannabis and CBD journey.

Another cost factor has to do with absorbability, which is quite low when CBD is swallowed. Ways of making it more absorbable to the body can also increase the cost, since these higher-tech formulations are expensive to make, though if it is truly a highly absorbably formula with data to back up that claim (check the product info) you would need to take less of it to get the same effect, so it may actually end up being cheaper in the end.

Different types of CBD products

The CBD products you see on the shelves at health shops in the UK and in most other places outside of a cannabis dispensary (legal in Canada and some US states) are hemp-based wellness products. These over-the-counter CBD products are derived from cannabis plants that are classified as hemp strains – meaning they contain less than 0.2% THC and can be legally cultivated in the UK and Europe. When people refer to CBD oil, this is the widely available type they are normally thinking of.

CBD is the same plant chemical whether it's from hemp varieties or from medical cannabis strains that are naturally higher in THC. However, even a small amount of THC may help make the CBD more effective for some people, especially when it comes to medical symptoms like severe chronic pain. Many people experiencing severe pain report needing much higher doses of hemp CBD oil with a maximum 0.2% THC content compared to taking a high-CBD medical cannabis oil by prescription with 1–2% THC. In some cases, the over-the-counter products may not work at all at the doses recommended. This is similar to other natural and also drug products that have an over-the-counter version as well as a stronger prescription version for when you need to bring out the big guns. However, for many wellness uses, over-the-counter hemp-based CBD oils work quite well, have virtually no side effects and can be bought without a prescription in the UK and the US. In Canada, all CBD products regardless of whether they are hemp-derived must be purchased at a licensed cannabis store with government ID and proof of age.

As mentioned above, the most important thing to find out about the product you choose is whether it's a full- or broad-spectrum product vs an isolate, so you know exactly what you are buying.

CBD isolate

CBD isolate is 99% pure CBD and lacks any other plant material, chlorophyll or other phytocannabinoids and terpenes. It does not have any smell and is tasteless, unlike full-spectrum CBD products, which smell to varying degrees slightly earthy due to the terpenes. It's generally considered a less effective form of CBD because it lacks the other plant chemicals that contribute to the entourage effect, helping to amplify the benefits of CBD. The upside of using CBD isolate is that it is easier to add to cosmetics, foods, etc. in a powder form, and in some preliminary studies at very high doses (600 mg) it may help lower feelings of anxiety. The issue is that generally with over-the-counter products you would have to take a whole bottle in one go to equal those study amounts.

CBD full-spectrum

CBD full-spectrum products are made from strains of the cannabis plant that fall into the hemp category but still contain other cannabinoids and terpenes in a full plant extract, meaning they have at least some level of the entourage effect. This is also called herbal synergy, where the plant chemicals all work together to act on our endocannabinoid system to a greater extent than CBD alone does, producing better effects at lower doses. A study done in mice looking at the difference between full-spectrum CBD vs CBD isolate revealed the same: CBD full-spectrum was superior to CBD isolate in reducing pain and inflammation.[2]

Most of my patients in Canada actually use high-CBD cannabis oils that contain 0.5%–1% THC. In the UK and the US, people generally use full-spectrum hemp CBD (which only contains 0.2% or less THC in the UK; 0.3% or less in the US), since prescription low-THC medical cannabis is hard to come by.

Some of the other minor cannabinoids found in a full-spectrum CBD product may include:

- cannabidiolic acid (CBDA)
- cannabidivarin (CBDV)
- cannabichromene (CBC)
- cannabigerol (CBG)
- cannabinol (CBN)

In addition, the most prominent terpenes in the oil should be listed on the product, although the exact amounts are often not reported, just shown as 'rich in X terpenes', such as:

- pinene
- myrcene
- beta-caryophyllene
- D-limonene

CBD broad-spectrum

Broad-spectrum CBD products are 'THC-free' – i.e. 0.00% THC (filtered out) – but have still retained at least some of their other plant chemicals, such as the cannabinoids, terpenes and flavonoids. In the UK, there is a movement towards THC-free products because some fear that any measurable THC in over-the-counter CBD products may not be allowed in the future, but at the time of writing, both were still on shelves. Broad-spectrum is the best choice for people who cannot have any THC residue (for example, athletes who got drug-tested, or in countries where any THC is still illegal or a grey zone).

Cannabis products containing over 0.2% (or 0.3%) THC

When we refer to products containing more than trace hemp levels of THC, this means any cannabis product of more than 0.2% (UK) or 0.3% (US) THC, normally about 1% THC or higher. Many of these products are still high in CBD too – there is a wide range of CBD and THC percentages and ratios available (more on that later in this chapter).

THC-containing cannabis medicines above the allowed hemp CBD product level are generally only available by prescription in most countries, if at all. This is the case in the UK. However, in Canada and some US states, these THC-containing products are now available to adults for recreational use without a prescription, just like alcohol. The shops that sell these products must have a licence, require government ID for proof of age and have strict guidelines on marketing to the public. This recreational cannabis use is regulated in a similar manner to alcohol and cigarette sales to prevent access to minors.

Cannabis medicines that are 'THC-rich' or high in THC are trickier to dose than hemp CBD products and should be tried slowly and cautiously, especially if you are new to THC. I believe THC should only be used under medical supervision if the purpose is for a health reason rather than a recreational one, as it is not without risk. However, it can be incredibly useful and therapeutic for many people and conditions, especially where their own endocannabinoid system may not be functioning normally.

The most well-known uses of THC are for severe pain, spasticity in neurological disorders, nausea from cancer treatments and insomnia. When prescribed cautiously and correctly, most patients report that they feel 'normal' and 'just good' but not high or impaired, especially if they get the right strain and dosage, which will be different for everyone. This is especially true in some of my patients with chronic fatigue syndrome and depression: a bit of THC, even in the daytime, can lift fatigue and sluggish depression symptoms, allowing them to function better. I have seen patients and clients with adult ADD/ADHD who had already tried self-medicating successfully with specific strains containing THC to help enhance their focus, reduce restlessness and 'sped-up thinking', and many preferred these over the prescription ADD medications. The effects on attention and focus appear to be very strain-dependent, at least in part. The ones that seem to work best in my experience are likely higher in pinene (reduces the temporary memory impairment from THC) and have more stimulating effects. They are often labelled as 'sativa' or 'daytime' strains and likely work on the dopamine circuits in some way.

Even if you choose a THC-rich product, I would almost always include CBD, which acts to reduce and buffer THC's potential side effects, such as increased heart rate, intoxication and anxiety/paranoia. This allows you to get the THC benefits with less risk of the downsides and minimal side effects in most cases.

The most important thing to remember when taking any cannabis medicine product is the 'start low, go slow' method. This means starting with what I would consider a micro dose, especially with anything that contains THC, and very slowly increasing it to the level that is right for you, which will differ from person to person because our endocannabinoid systems are all slightly different. Like many other whole-plant botanical medicines, CBD and cannabis are to a large extent self-guided and self-titrated (which means the patient slowly increases their dose each day or every few days by a specific tiny amount), but having some guidelines to help direct you makes it much easier and more successful.

I have also found over the years that the very high doses (especially with CBD) used in research studies and clinical trials are often not needed in order to see a benefit – it's a case of the published research not matching up with my clinical experience of thousands of people, and is something I have heard from my colleagues who also prescribe CBD and cannabis. There are many possible reasons for this: individual variation, absorption differences, the type of product used in the studies (often a CBD isolate or isolated THC vs a natural full- or broad-spectrum CBD or cannabis oil) and also the strains chosen. That being said, some people may need more than the average dose. It's a process of personal exploration guided by a tried-and-tested method I've found helpful over the years for my patients and clients.

I will go into detail about caveats and cautions about cannabis in the next chapter, so make sure you read that before experimenting, but first let's dive into how to choose a product and how to take it.

Forms of cannabis and CBD

Cannabis is a unique botanical medicine in that it can be used effectively in many ways: topically for skin conditions, transdermally in a patch to work through the body in a slow-release form, taken in a pill form or as an oil by mouth or in a tincture, sublingually (under the tongue), and even rectally or vaginally in some specific cases for issues such as period pain or gut problems. It can also be inhaled via vaporisation, similarly to an asthma inhaler in some cases, or in other cases closer to an e-cigarette.

There are many factors that go into which form and way of taking CBD may be best for you. The most common way to take it currently is in an oral oil or capsule, but a lot of people also find vaporising cannabis is very effective for them – or in many cases, using a combination of these methods. Less popular methods but that have higher absorbablity and last longer, such as transdermal patches, may become more popular as more of these 'high-tech' products become available as a solution to the low absorbablity issue. In the chapters that follow, I will give additional tips and suggestions to help guide how you may want to start incorporating CBD wellness products and/ or medical cannabis (where it is legal and with your doctor's help!) into your life.

First I'll give you a practical explanation of each mode of use and some examples of when it may be best used.

Sublingual tinctures, sprays and lozenges

Tinctures have been used for thousands of years in herbal medicine and may have been one of the earliest cannabis medicines apart from smoking. They are made by soaking the cannabis or CBD flower in alcohol or, for alcohol-free glycerine-based tinctures, by a process called hydrolysis using high pressures. This way of taking a CBD or cannabis product may allow you to get slightly better absorption than an edible or a capsule because the spray or tincture drops are dosed under the tongue (sublingually) and some may be absorbed directly through the skin on the inside of the mouth, which is rich in tiny blood vessels. However, the issue still remains that even with under the tongue dosing, because CBD and cannabinoids are 'fat loving' they don't absorb easily via the mouth or oral route.

Lozenges are solid, like boiled sweets, and are meant to be dissolved slowly under the tongue for sublingual absorption, just like a spray or tincture but on a slower release. The absorbability will probably vary between different lozenges.

Most of the products on the shelves currently are not in a tincture or sublingual form but are sold as oral oils, since this is the way they are most commonly produced for bigger batches most cost effectively.

Oral ingestion

Cannabis and CBD products that are swallowed or ingested all pass through the gut and go to the liver to get broken down. This process is called the first-pass effect, and it means that less of the active cannabinoids like CBD and THC get directly into the bloodstream, even less so than sublingual tinctures and lozenges. Oral ways of using cannabis are normally broken down into four categories:

1. CBD and cannabis oil. Hemp-based CBD oil is the most common product you will come across without a prescription, especially from health shops and online. It is one of the most accessible and safest ways to start using a CBD or cannabis medicine product. Taking the oil with a meal or a snack containing fat (e.g. a spoonful of nut butter), since CBD is 'fat loving', may slightly increase how well it is absorbed, but there are not studies yet to prove this.

2. Capsules. The upside of capsules is that they are very easy to take, have no scent, are discreet (no one has to know it's cannabis, as it looks like any other supplement) and you also know exactly the dose of CBD and THC you're getting, as it

must be stated on the bottle. However, they pass through the digestive system first so do not have any sublingual absorption in the mouth.

3. Gummies (gummy bears). CBD gummies are becoming more popular, as are cannabis gummies containing THC in Canada and some US states where recreational cannabis is legal without a prescription. CBD gummies and THC cannabis gummies both go through the digestive system, and are usually labelled with the exact amount of CBD/THC per gummy. Although technically they are a form of edible, I think of them as slightly different, since with edibles the recipe is usually in bulk and you don't know the exact amount of cannabinoids in each serving. Hemp CBD gummies may contain sugar and are often very low dose, and some are made from CBD isolate so may be less effective as a wellness or health-use form.

4. Edibles. For wellness and medical uses, edibles such as brownies, cookies and cannabis butter spread on bread or crackers are my least favourite method because it's almost impossible to dose them accurately, and the absorption amounts and duration of the effects (especially important with THC-containing edibles!) are unpredictable and erratic. That is not an issue if you use hemp-based CBD oil in an edible, because putting in twice the amount won't harm you or make you feel high; it may just lead to a very expensive brownie batch! The CBD brownies often found in cafés and snack bars are normally quite low-potency and definitely won't hurt you – you can think of them the same way as having a turmeric latte. The potential safety issue is with THC-containing edibles because the batch-to-batch variation means that it is not uncommon to misdose and end up feeling intoxicated – exactly what my medical cannabis patients are trying to avoid! Cannabis edibles can also be mistaken for normal brownies or gummy bears, so keeping them locked away from kids to avoid accidental ingestion is very important.

HOW MUCH CBD OIL IS ACTUALLY GETTING ABSORBED INTO THE BLOODSTREAM?

It is often recommended that CBD and cannabis oils taken orally should be held under the tongue so they get partly absorbed through the small blood vessels in the mucosa, or skin lining, and reach the bloodstream more directly before they are swallowed. This is a good tip to try, but unless it is a special sublingual preparation in a high-tech system, some of the oil will still have to pass through the digestive system before ending up in the bloodstream.

How much actually gets absorbed into the blood varies between products, based on factors such as whether the CBD is encapsulated, or made in a high-tech process (such as liposomal CBD, or vesicle technology, or some method of microencapsulation). The more high-tech the product is, the higher the price tag generally. However, as discussed previously, the benefit may be getting higher absorption for lower amounts, meaning you need to take much less to get the same effect. The tricky thing is that there are many products that claim to enhance the bioavailability of CBD without any proof of the technology they use – it may not be what they say it is – especially online, many unproven claims exist. That being said, there are other supplements (and drugs) that have been developed and tested in preliminary studies using a high-tech method to enhance their absorbability in the body, and the same can be done with CBD and cannabinoids. If it truly is what it says it is, it is likely worth the higher price tag if the difference means you have to use a fraction of the amount. If you want to dip your toe in the water of CBD, then choosing a cheaper but still good-quality tested product may be the way to go first, as many people find they benefit from these too as part of their wellness supplement regimen daily. Then if you want more bang for your buck, look for a higher tech product with a proven delivery system.   »

» There is also individual variation in how fast people metabolise something, or break it down in the liver with special enzymes that vary slightly from person to person. Taking your CBD oil with a meal may also increase the absorption, or bioavailability, since it is best absorbed with fats.[3]

Oral cannabis products (capsules, oils and gummies) that are not in high-tech carrier systems are estimated to have bioavailability between 6 and 10%,[4] which is pretty low but still has an effect for many. In addition, a greater percentage of the oil taken may interact with special receptors in the gut wall before it is absorbed through the gut lining, and this may also contribute to its effect, but at the time of writing, this is only still a theory. This may be the case with terpenes from cannabis too, not just CBD: they are in such low concentrations in the blood they are barely detectable but may work via gut interactions. We are still learning the details of all the ways cannabis and CBD work in the body. Cannabinoids are lipophilic (fat-loving, water-hating), and don't dissolve well in body fluids and in the bloodstream, but build up instead in places like our fat cells and can get released back into the bloodstream slowly over time, making measuring levels of cannabinoids in the body tricky.

Topicals

Topicals are products that you apply on the top of the skin. This includes everything from lip balms to anti-ageing and acne creams, as well as body lotions and body butters and salves for pain. The way topical products are made varies widely, as does the absorption and efficacy; high-tech formulas with liposomes, nanoparticles or encapsulated ingredients may help penetrate the skin to a greater extent. One ingredient type to look out for is terpenes such as linalool and limonene, as these may enhance penetration. Linalool and limonene are naturally found in cannabis, as well as in lavender and citrus fruits.

Menthol is another helpful terpene, found in cannabis as well as in many varieties of mint.

When it comes to using both CBD and cannabis topicals containing THC (generally only available through prescription or some dispensaries in the US and Canada), it is hard to overdo it – they are extremely safe, and using a topical balm with CBD and THC won't make you high or cause you to feel intoxicated. This is one of the most common concerns people have when they first try a cannabis- or even a hemp-based CBD topical. When I was given my first cannabis topical salve after my hand injury, I knew logically that it would not make me high or impair me even though it had some THC in it, but I had a barely conscious fear around it based on my years of anti-cannabis conditioning. However, after using a topical cream liberally six times a day, I discovered for myself that it was definitely not impairing or intoxicating in any way. That being said, if you are drug-tested for your work or you are a professional athlete and use a product with ingredients to help penetrate the deeper layers of the skin and possibly reach the bloodstream, it is advisable to stay away from topicals that contain THC, since this may be a banned substance in some workplaces and sports federations.

Transdermal patches

Transdermal patches are used to deliver cannabinoids systemically (meaning throughout the brain and body) via the bloodstream. They use a patch that looks like a plaster stuck onto the skin, but contains a specialised formula to penetrate past the skin into the bloodstream. In this way they are unlike a topical cream or salve, which is used for local pain relief or for a skin effect such as anti-acne. These patches can contain just CBD from hemp (available without a prescription in the UK just like CBD oil) or CBD and THC, or mainly THC (the latter being for medical cannabis with a doctor's prescription). They use specialised high-tech methods to help the CBD (and THC if by prescription) penetrate the skin and reach the bloodstream to deliver the cannabinoids straight into the circulation, and are designed for slow release of CBD and/or THC as a highly absorbable alternative to oral or sublingual cannabis and/or vaporising for people who want a systemic effect.

They work in a similar way to prescription pain patches, only with cannabinoids rather than painkillers inside the patch. Nicotine patches and birth control contraceptive patches are similar too, in that they are stuck onto the skin using the same technology with the active ingredients absorbed systemically throughout the bloodstream. The cool thing is that this drug technology can be used to deliver natural cannabinoids and CBD too, although it hasn't yet hit the mainstream. Because this method is a highly absorbable way of using CBD, I believe it will become more and more popular and may even eventually take over from CBD oil as a preferred method of CBD use, as well as for cannabis medicine by prescription. This method also avoids having to go through the digestive system first, leading to more active cannabinoids and terpenes being delivered directly into the bloodstream. Terpenes are also easily broken down in the gut, so this may offer the best way to get a wider spectrum of plant chemicals into the blood apart from vaporising and inhaling it multiple times a day.

Vaginal

This method was used traditionally for thousands of years according to some ancient texts, including in ancient Egypt,[5] for pain in childbirth and helping with labour. More recently, some companies have started making 'CBD tampons' and users claim that they have found them helpful for period pain. Although studies proving this are lacking, I find I am constantly asked by journalists to comment on this use. It is not a way I currently prescribe CBD or cannabis in my medical practice, as it is a very little studied area so far.

However, I have spoken to many women who have tried products such as CBD vaginal inserts and think it has helped their period pain. Often, they report, it helped as much or more so than other things they had tried including pain pills. So that is the beginning of some anecdotal evidence at least! It may be worth experimenting with if someone requires high doses of strong painkillers or anti-inflammatories every month to cope with their painful period symptoms. Hopefully we will soon have some more research to shed further light on this interesting usage. I'm intrigued! I can theorise that CBD may exert local anti-inflammatory properties, and maybe it is this that is helping with menstrual discomfort and pain. So far, there are no reports to my knowledge of CBD increasing the risk of TSS (toxic shock syndrome) above that of normal tampon use so so far, so good.

Other companies are focusing on developing CBD- (and where legal, THC-) infused personal lubricants to enhance sexual pleasure, and vaginal suppositories to aid with menstrual cramping and pain. Again, there are currently no published research studies in this area, but it appears that many women are starting to try vaginal CBD for themselves as a likely low-risk intervention for menstrual pain.

Rectal

Similar to vaginal applications for women, rectal suppositories containing cannabis may have been used traditionally to treat conditions of the bowel and anal fissures in both men and women for hundreds and possibly even thousands of years, but it is hard to say exactly how they were used and at what doses. There are no controlled published studies in humans on the absorption, uptake and effects of THC, CBD and other cannabinoids via the rectal suppository route. Despite this, many people have tried rectal suppositories with either CBD alone or a combination of both CBD and THC, and report good results. One study in rats reported that rectal CBD decreased colon inflammation, but so far that's all the published research we have.

THC on its own is not absorbed rectally, so most patients report they do not get high or intoxicated by using THC capsules in this way. However, I have seen cases where very large amounts of THC rectally *did* cause feelings of slight intoxication, so it remains an unknown exactly how much can be taken and how individual differences may factor in. A new 'pre-form' of THC is being tested[6] for rectal administration in small preliminary human studies. It has been successful in getting THC into the bloodstream but it's not yet available outside of a research lab at the time of writing. When it does become available, it may be great news for patients with nausea and vomiting, where THC can be very helpful but they cannot keep anything down by mouth.

Vaporised CBD and cannabis

Dried CBD flowers from hemp (containing less than 0.2/0.3% THC) can be purchased in some locations, but currently in the UK it is technically not legal to sell even hemp CBD flowers. In Canada and some US states, cannabis flowers that contain THC are available by prescription, as well as without a prescription from special stores that sell cannabis for legal recreational use. These dried flowers (or buds, as they are often known in the non-medical world) are traditionally the form of cannabis many people think of when it comes to what is rolled to smoke in a joint. However, for medical or wellness use, smoking cannabis or CBD flower is not recommended, as it may be unsafe for the lungs due to the burning of the plant material. Potential risks may include an increased likelihood of lung cancer (though the evidence on this is conflicted). This cancer risk appears much lower than that associated with smoking cigarettes or even self-rolled tobacco leaves, and this is thought to be due to the many anti-inflammatory and anti-cancer chemicals in cannabis that may counteract the harmful effects of inhaling burned material.

If an inhaled route is preferred, it is recommended instead to use a high-quality herbal vaporiser to gently heat the dried plant material. This allows the vapours containing the medicinal plant chemicals (CBD, THC, minor cannabinoids and terpenes) to vaporise off the plant without burning it. It is very important if you are going to inhale cannabis flower product to ensure it has been tested for moulds, biotoxins and contaminants, as inhaling these may lead to serious health issues and side effects (see end of this chapter for how to choose a safe product).

I have many patients who are ex-cigarette smokers, and in many cases they prefer to avoid using a vaporiser for fear of triggering a smoking craving. If you are also an ex-smoker, you may want to consider a different method of CBD delivery. For people who are currently trying to quit smoking or change from nicotine e-cigarettes, however, CBD vaporising can be a good option, safer and non-addictive, and may reduce anxiety, which is a symptom that often worsens in nicotine withdrawal.

Vaporising is the quickest way of getting cannabis and cannabinoids like CBD (and THC, depending on the type of flower used) as well as terpenes into the bloodstream and to the brain to work their magic. In other words, it is an immediate-release and highly absorbable form of cannabis.

One caveat to using a vaporised THC-containing product is that because it works so quickly and reaches the brain within minutes, it also has a higher chance of causing a feeling of intoxication, especially if you are new to THC or the dose was too high for your tolerance level. It may also lead to other temporary THC side effects such as rapid heart rate, dysphoria and even paranoia and anxiety. This is dose-dependent, however, and usually avoidable by using a flower that also contains lots of CBD to buffer these effects. Use a very tiny amount at a time until you are adjusted, and then work with your medical practitioner on titrating your dose and monitoring for side effects. Of my patients who had previously had a negative experience with self-medication or recreational use of cannabis, it was often as a result of smoking or vaporising a very high-THC, low-CBD strain in large amounts, something we do not recommend for wellness or medical use.

How to use vaporised CBD and cannabis flowers

The dose needed will vary from person to person depending on whether you are new to cannabis or have been using it regularly, the strain and percentage of THC and CBD in the flower chosen, and how deep and long you inhale. If you start using one strain and find your ideal dose, but then change to a different strain, or even the same strain but grown by a different company or in slightly different conditions, which may change the cannabinoid and terpene profile, you might need to adjust your dose, so always use the 'start low, go slow' approach when changing strains or suppliers. If you are using a hemp CBD flower with only trace THC, overdoing it is not an issue, so you can be quite liberal with the amounts you use, but just to be safe, always start with the smallest amount and then add from there!

- Start with one matchstick-head-sized amount of ground-up flower (see below for how to grind it and prepare it for the vaporiser). As time goes on, you can increase the amount you use per session to your preference.
- Take one 3-second-long inhalation, hold for 1–2 seconds and then exhale.
- After the first inhalation, wait 5–15 minutes before taking a second (err on the longer end of range if you are cannabis-naive or if there are any relative risk factors present, such as cardiac risk factors). If you are using a flower with THC and you are new to cannabis, wait a full 15 minutes before taking a second inhaled dose. If you are used to it, you may want to take a second dose as soon as 5 minutes later if you have not yet felt any effect on the symptom you are targeting.
- Record your response after 5–10 minutes, i.e. self-assess the response in a tracker or symptom journal that you will review with your doctor (e.g. is the pain or other symptom better, worse or the same?).
- Continue inhalations spread out at least 5–10 minutes apart until you reach the desired effect or you start to experience a side effect (only an issue with THC flowers), such as accelerated heart rate, anxiety, etc.
- For medical cannabis patients who use vaporised cannabis products by prescription, generally between 0.5 and 1 g/day is enough, and many people use far less than this. I have some patients who only use about 0.1–0.2 g/day of vaporised flower

plus a high-CBD oil to manage symptoms like fatigue, low mood or anxiety on an as-needed basis, and this approach has been very effective.

General guidance on vaporising

Keep the temperature setting on the vaporiser under 217°C to avoid boiling off toxic naphthalene, which occurs at this temperature and higher. Start your inhalations at between 185 and 201°C – you can test different temperatures, as there is much variation. The temperature variations affect which cannabinoids get vaporised off preferentially, since each of the 160 cannabinoids plus each of the terpenes boils off at a slightly different temperature. So even if you use the same flower material but you choose a different temperature, you may notice a slightly altered feeling or effect. For example, THC boils off at 157°C, while CBD starts at 160 and ends at 180°C. CBN, a breakdown product of THC, which also tends to have pain-relieving and sedating or calming properties, boils off even higher, at 185°C.

Vaporising cannabis, as well as CBD hemp flowers, will produce a smell and taste, both of which come from the plant terpenes. These will be slightly different for each strain. Some people are very sensitive to the smell or taste of cannabis, and some strains are more pungent than others. It is a very individual preference. Some can smell and taste citrusy or even fruity, while others can have a smell that some would call skunky or earthy. If you try a strain and cannot stand the smell or taste, try changing to a different strain until you find one you like. The terpene make-up that changes the smell and taste can also change the strain's effects. So the bottom line is: don't give up on all vaporised cannabis if the first one you try does not agree with you smell- and taste-wise.

Avoid using untested street cannabis for vaporising. This is because multiple sample analysis studies of street cannabis have shown evidence of contaminants such as ammonia, chemicals and pesticide residues, or even illegal drugs such as cocaine and synthetic cannabis, known as 'spice'. It is impossible to be sure of the origin or growing methods of cannabis purchased on the black market.

Street cannabis is often produced by unsafe methods, the main purpose being selling it to people who want to feel high, not use it for wellness or health purposes.

> ## NOTE ON E-CIGARETTE-STYLE VAPORISERS AND VAPE LIQUIDS
>
> Some oil-based vape pens with cannabis isolates may contain other chemicals that may be unsafe to inhale, such as propylene glycol (which when heated may convert to formaldehyde). Other contaminants of concern, especially with black market THC vapes, include a natural additive called vitamin E acetate, which may cause a serious, even life-threatening, lung reaction in some people. Legal CBD vapes are not allowed to contain this vitamin E acetate so they are safer. For now, I find the best effects come from using the actual cannabis plant material (flower) in a dried herbal vaporiser. However, new vaporised cannabis high-tech delivery systems are currently in the research and development stages and starting to appear in shops in North America. These may allow full-spectrum CBD and cannabis to be vaporised in a measured dose without having to use the actual dried plant material, while also avoiding the potential risks of vape pens containing chemical additives.

Instructions for using a dried herbal vaporiser

- Grind the dry flower using a stainless-steel, non-coated hand grinder, or one made from hemp, which is my favourite.
- Pack the chamber of the vaporiser by scooping the ground flower into the chamber, starting with a matchstick-head-sized amount.
- Set the temperature. Normally this is on the side of the device, although some brands will do it via an app on your phone that is paired with the device via Bluetooth. Try experimenting between 185°C and 201°C.
- Try to inhale for the same number of seconds each time to estimate the dose as accurately as possible.

- After each session, clean the chamber and the mouthpiece using the brush for your device.

> ### THE FUTURE OF VAPORISING CBD AND CANNABIS
>
> A few companies in the US and Israel are working on asthma-inhaler vaporisers that offer an exact dosage of CBD and THC via inhalation. This would overcome the issue of accurately measuring precise dosages with current vaporisers. These new vaporisers are pre-loaded with dried cannabis flower pressed into a pellet or an ampoule containing full-spectrum vaporised cannabis. They would be easy to use for patients who may have disabilities, weakness, poor dexterity, tremors or poor vision and may revolutionise the vaporising delivery system for cannabis medicines but are still in the research stages at the time of writing and likely to be very expensive at least for a while to come.

How to choose a suitable dried herb vaporiser

There are two main types of dried herb vaporisers. No matter which type you choose, pick a brand and product with a warranty if you can, as these are an investment of £100 or more so you want to make sure it lasts.

Conduction-only vaporisers are the most common type. They heat the flower via direct contact with a heating element. Some brands can be simple to use, as they have fewer buttons, but not all. According to users, conduction-only vaporisers tend to use up the flower product more quickly and don't heat plant material as evenly, but there are a few options in this category that are very easy to use, such as the Pax 3, one of my favourites.

Convection/conduction mixed-type vaporisers don't offer as many brands and options, but some people prefer this type. They heat the ground-up plant material evenly as you inhale, and some claim this helps preserve the terpenes, though no actual studies confirm this!

It may make each batch of cannabis dried flower last longer and improve the taste, but again this is subjective. My favourites from this category are the Lynx Gaia and the Mighty, which is bulkier, designed more for medical use, with a chamber that is easy to fill.

WHAT IS KIEF?

Kief is the crystal-like powdery and sticky substance that naturally exudes from the resin glands on the cannabis flower trichomes and, to a lesser extent, the leaves. This can be compressed into hashish blocks, or in some cases sprinkled on top of CBD or cannabis flower in a dried herbal vaporiser to increase the effects and potency. Like the flower, it is difficult to dose exactly (in fact it is harder!). It is not a common CBD or medical cannabis product, but is more commonly found in recreational shops in places where they are legal. Kief is often extremely high in THC.

Dosing information for hemp-based CBD wellness products

With CBD wellness products that are ingested, there is no single right dose for every person and use. The optimal dose may also vary from product to product, depending on the other minor cannabinoids and terpenes present as well as whether it's a high-tech formulation, even if the amount of CBD is the same, as we discussed earlier. That makes giving a general dosing guide for all products together very difficult. Everyone's endocannabinoid system and response to CBD is also different, because we are each unique. If we are in a stressed, out-of-balance state, the response to a product may be different to when we are calm, centred and stress-free, perhaps after a relaxing holiday. So even in the same person, the optimal dose can change depending on other life factors, because we are dynamic beings in constant flux.

Because hemp CBD products are so safe (as long as they do not contain contaminants), there is no such thing as overdosing on CBD.

That being said, starting at a relatively small dose is generally rec-ommended. People who respond at low doses will be pleasantly surprised by how much money it can save them if a small dose is sufficient. It's not a case of taking it for a month and stopping and then expecting it to have permanently cured a symptom or issue. I have found with my patients that you need to keep at it, taking CBD regularly for 3–6 months in some cases to see a significant effect, or to keep gaining benefit even if you have already noticed a difference after a week or two (it is common with things like anxiety or stress to see a return quite quickly). However, some people do find they just use it when they are going through a stressful period to help give them a bit of an extra booster, and in this case using a higher dose to get a quicker benefit may be worthwhile.

Note on dosing for each chapter

For each chapter, the general dosing guidelines are based on non-high-tech regular CBD oil and medical cannabis oil products, which have been around the longest. However, as the science of CBD and cannabis advances, we are likely to see more and more novel delivery systems for CBD. These products will likely enhance absorption and even bioavailablity by a huge amount, meaning you need to take less of it. Some new forms will also provide long-acting slow release of CBD and cannabis into the bloodstream to help avoid issues with the highs and lows of immediate-release dosing, just like we can now do with many other drugs as well as other natural botanicals and nutra-ceuticals. These are not widely available yet at the time of writing but are likely to become more common and more affordable as time goes on alongside traditional CBD oils, and may represent the 'second wave' of CBD and medical cannabis. These new shifts may change the average dose amounts to some extent, but regardless, the 'start low, go slow' approach will still hold true for any product you wish to try.

If you are extremely sensitive to any supplements, foods, drugs or over-the-counter remedies or you suffer with multiple chemical sensitivities, you may want to start with the micro or ultra-low dose. However, for most people, the average starting dose is fine.

Micro or ultra-low starting dose for CBD oil: 5 mg 2x/day with a meal.

Average starting dose for CBD oil: 10 mg 2–3x/day with a meal.

Stay at the first dose for 3–4 days, then increase by 1–2 mg/dose. Stay at that new dose for another 2 days, and monitor response in a journal or tracker: pain, anxiety, stress, energy, etc. If no response, continue to increase dose in the same way (1–2 mg/dose) every few days until a response is seen for the issue you are trying to target. If you are just using CBD for general wellness, you can track things like stress level, mood and sleep quality as a marker of how it's going, keeping in mind that changes may be subtle.

With CBD wellness products as well as medical cannabis oils by prescription, the longer people stick with them and use them on a daily basis, the better results they tend to get, especially if they are using it for a chronic symptom like pain or anxiety. I find this is especially true with hemp CBD products (with only trace THC). You may not feel anything immediately after taking your CBD. However, over a period of weeks and months, when used daily, and slowly increasing the dose, people often start to notice improvements with issues such as headaches, stress, anxiety, problems getting to sleep, and body aches and pains, even when they have not made any other lifestyle or supplement changes.

Some people may end up taking 25–30 mg/day of CBD, while others find they do best at 60 or even 80 mg/day. For the purposes of this book, these doses are for the average good-quality CBD oil since this is still the most common form you will see on the shelves at the time of writing. For potent anti-inflammatory effects, going as high as 200 mg/day can be beneficial, and even higher when using CBD under medical supervision in the treatment of seizures. It really depends on you, your symptoms and their severity, what else is going on in your life and your unique make-up. Some people find that when they are feeling good and not under too much stress, the lower dose helps to keep them well. During times of increased stress or an injury or lack of sleep, they may need to take a bit more. You can adjust your dose up and down as stress levels and symptoms fluctuate naturally over time. As a caveat, some bodies such as the FCA in the UK have recently recommended that healthy adults do not exceed 70 mg/day of CBD and that anyone taking a medication should not take CBD at all. The recommendation comes from a COT (Comittee on Toxicity) recent review although I am still unclear as to the 'data' that went into their decision as, curiously, I am not aware of any human good-quality data that CBD is unsafe in the amounts suggested for most people and certainly clinically I have not come across this. However, it is important for consumers to be aware of such advice. In the US, the FDA still does not consider CBD to meet its requirements to be classified/sold/marketed as a supplement, although this may change in the future.

Taking CBD will not magically make all of your problems go away overnight – no supplement on earth can do that, no matter what the marketing may tell you! However, CBD wellness products can be incredibly useful tools for a busy, hectic lifestyle as part of your self-care regimen.

How long does CBD stay in my system?

The research is still at quite an early stage in humans, but preliminary studies suggest that for a single dose of CBD taken by mouth, the half-life is 1–2 days. A half-life is the amount of time it takes for half of the dose to be eliminated from the body. This is just an estimate, as everyone will be slightly different depending on their metabolism or how fast or slow their unique enzymes break down substances. Also, as we've learned, because cannabinoids are fat-loving, they build up in the body's fatty tissues over time if you use them daily or regularly.[7,8]

Dosing information for products containing medical cannabis

When using any products containing THC above the trace amounts found in hemp CBD, we employ a method called 'start low, go slow'. What this means is that we start at a very low micro dose, work slowly up to the optimal dose over a period of 6–8 weeks and then reassess for another few weeks at that dose. This method is not one-size- or one-dose-fits-all; it's very much a self-led self-titration method based on some guidelines that I have found useful when working with thousands of patients using products containing THC.

I also find that because everyone's system is unique, it is important to use this opportunity of starting medical cannabis to get in tune with your body and brain. Reconnecting to our body's intuition is so important, and something that many Western medicine doctors unfortunately discourage or sometimes even laugh at. This process of self-discovery and intuition about what feels right for your body is incredibly powerful and empowering, especially if you have suffered from a poorly understood chronic condition or have had multiple Western medicine failures for your chronic symptoms. You may also discover that it is hard to find a medical doctor who is a true expert in medical cannabis and botanical medicine. Even some of the doctors who prescribe cannabis are not experts in its use. Ideally you will work closely with a doctor or practitioner with an open mind who is willing to go on the journey of self-discovery with you, even if they are not yet an expert. You will quickly become your own expert, not just in cannabis but in your body and its needs. These dosing guidelines are for a non-high-tech cannabis oil or capsule containing the cannabis oil inside of it. For vaporised cannabis dosing, see the section above.

Micro or ultra-low starting dose for THC: 1 mg an hour before bed.

Average starting dose for THC: 2 mg an hour before bed.

Daytime

- Start with a high-CBD, low-THC oil (10–18% CBD, 0.5–2% THC, or an approximate ratio of 20–25:1).
- Starting dose: 5 mg 2–3x/day (a.m./lunchtime/before bed); increase every 4–5 days by 1–2 mg each dose.
- Monitor response in a journal or tracker: pain, anxiety, stress, energy, etc. If no response, continue to increase dose in the same way (1–2 mg/dose) every few days until a response is seen for the issue you are trying to target.
- Try to take consistently with food to enhance absorption.

- Avoid any high-THC oils or high-THC products during the daytime if you are not used to them.

Night-time

- Start with 1–2 mg of a high-THC indica-dominant oil if needed to help with severe night-time pain or insomnia. Taking before sleep will help you to habituate to the effects of THC so that you do not feel intoxicated or impaired during the daytime.
- Increase by 1–2 mg every few days until pain relief or sleep benefit is achieved or potential THC side effects become an issue (such as feeling hung-over in the morning, dizziness, lethargy, increased heart rate or palpitations).
- The optimal dose is variable from person to person and depends on many factors, including symptom severity, other medications, sleep dysfunction and individual variation in the way your brain and body processes THC. Many people work up to their effective dose of 10 mg or less, while others with more severe symptoms may need 15–20 mg (built up to over a period of approximately six weeks).
- Newer forms of dosing such as transdermal medical cannabis and CBD patches may allow for dosing only every few days with continuous slow release, and lower risk of side effects and needing very high oral oil doses in some people to get desired effects but this is not yet the standard form available.

The above recommendations are for people new to cannabis and THC. Experienced patients may be able to tolerate more daytime THC, especially if they have severe daytime pain, without feeling impaired. In these cases, I will sometimes add more daytime THC after 2–4 weeks of getting them used to THC at night first. This can be done by using a daytime cannabis oil that has a more balanced CBD to THC ratio (5:1 or even 1:1) in place of the high-CBD oil. Another option is to keep the high-CBD oil (20–25:1) as the base for the daytime and add inhaled cannabis with THC for breakthrough symptoms like pain and fatigue. This option is good if people need to drive later in the day, so that they can vaporise in the morning for symptom relief but not feel impaired a few hours later. Vaporised cannabis wears off faster than the ingested oils or capsules or sublingual tinctures, which can last much or even most of the day. In general, the goal is to keep the CBD to THC ratio high initially and to use the smallest effective dose of THC needed to control symptoms.

If a patient reports already using a self-medication dosage of approximately 2 g/day of high-THC street cannabis, smoked, I may transition them on to medical cannabis in the following way:

- Base of therapy for daytime: start with 10–15 mg 3x/day (morning, noon, 5 p.m.) of high-CBD, low-THC oil or capsule and titrate up.
- Night-time (if sleep is disrupted): 5 mg before bed of THC in oil or capsule form, titrate slowly to symptom relief/side effect.
- Vaporising: a balanced THC/CBD strain, one for daytime and one possibly a bit higher in THC for evening pain/symptoms and getting to sleep in the amount of 0.5–1 g/day to start.

How long does THC stay in my system?

The half-life of THC varies from person to person and also seems based on how often you use THC. The more often you take it, the more it builds up, and the longer it takes for the body to get rid of it. The half-life can vary between 4 and 12 days. If you use THC very regularly, it is possible there will still be some left in your system even after 30 days. This is a consideration if you have to take a drug test for cannabis (which normally means they are looking for THC).[9]

What to do if you have (or may have had) a THC side effect

For most people, the side effects of THC, such as increased heart rate and feeling intoxicated, are dose-dependent and usually minimal when taken under medical supervision using the 'start low, go slow' approach. This is generally the case as long as you start at the recommended dose and increase it very slowly, as well as ensuring you are taking a product that contains at least an even ratio of CBD to THC. If side effects occur initially, they tend to go away as tolerance develops over a 2–4-week period. This topic is discussed in detail in Chapter Six, but the most common side effects with THC are: increased heart rate, anxiety, intoxication, dry mouth or dry eyes and dizziness.

Luckily, the beneficial effects of THC on symptoms such as pain, spasm and sleep do not tend to taper off when you become tolerant to the side effects. The benefits are usually sustained without needing bigger and bigger doses once the optimal dose is reached. If you have a heart condition, however, or certain other medical issues, or if others in your family have them, THC may not be safe for you at all, or only in very small doses under strict medical supervision. To make sure that's not you, please read Chapter Six before trying anything (and of course, even then always consult with your doctor to see what is right for you).

If you take a cannabis oil containing THC for night-time pain and/or insomnia and you experience a side effect, there are three good options:

1. For your next time, reduce the dose to the previous dose that you tolerated before experiencing the side effect. Stay at that dose for 3–5 days and reassess before increasing again.
2. Increase the amount of CBD taken with your THC oil to buffer the THC side effects. For example, if you are using an oil that has a 1:10 ratio of CBD to THC, add a hemp-based CBD or very low-THC (0.5%), high-CBD oil to your THC-containing product dose (e.g. if you are taking a 5 mg THC dose using the 1:10 high-THC oil before bed, stay at this dose but add from a second bottle an additional 10 mg or more of CBD).
3. If the side effect you experienced was a feeling of morning grogginess or slight hangover, but you otherwise slept well and had a good response for symptom relief overnight, you can try taking the oil an hour earlier so it wears off before you wake up.

You can also try adding a THC herbal antidote to your daily regimen, which some people self-report has helped, although there are no published research studies for this trick yet, such as:

- Lemon juice – cold as lemonade.
- Peppercorn – can be sprinkled onto food or added to turmeric powder or juice as a hot latte.
- Calamus root tincture – this herbal medicine has anti-anxiety, relaxant and laxative properties, and was thought to have been used in ancient Egypt as well as in traditional Indian herbal medicine (Ayurveda) where it is mixed with cannabis. According to Indian traditional texts, it is thought to block or neutralise some of the intoxicant effects of cannabis.[10,11]

How to read a lab test for a product

Because cannabis is a soil-cleaning plant, it can suck up all sorts of bad stuff, especially if grown outdoors in a contaminated area. The best practice whenever possible is to try to choose products that have been tested by a third-party or independent lab. This makes sure the testing is unbiased, and any product that has gone through the process will have a certificate of analysis (COA) so you know that it does what is says on the tin (and doesn't have anything extra you don't want, like contaminants or heavy metals!). A COA is only given to accredited (i.e. legitimate) testing labs. These can vary in name depending on what country you are in, but in the UK this type of lab is called an 'accredited ISO 17025 analytical laboratory'.

These labs must use equipment and methods that have been validated for testing cannabinoids, such as a technique known as high-performance liquid chromatography (HPLC), which is known as the industry standard for testing CBD wellness and medical cannabis products. There is an even better method, called ultra-performance liquid chromatography (UPLC), but it is more expensive and not as commonly used. To test for terpenes, most experts agree that standard HPLC is not the best or most accurate method, and another technique called gas chromatography (GC) is recommended instead, although not all labs can perform this.

The lab report, aka the COA, should contain the following information:

CBD content

CBD oil and any over-the-counter CBD products should have accurate reporting on CBD content per bottle/ml/capsule, depending on the form of the product. For example, if a product says on the label that it contains 500 mg of CBD in a 30 ml bottle, that would give you approximately 17 mg of CBD per 1 ml. This is known as the reported value. In the COA report, the value found by the third-party lab needs to be within 10% of that reported value on the product label.

So to see how much CBD you will get per serving if the dropper the product comes with is 1 ml, you divide the total CBD amount in the bottle by the number of millilitres to get the amount per dose (in this example 500 mg/30 = 16.66 mg CBD/dropperful).

THC content

For both hemp CBD wellness products and medical cannabis products, accurate THC content should be listed, even if it is a THC-free product. Many CBD wellness products have been found upon testing to contain significant amounts of THC, although they were initially labelled as hemp. For hemp CBD wellness products, the THC reported should be 0.2% or lower, which is not nearly enough to cause intoxication at normal doses (i.e. unless you guzzled 10 bottles in one go and even then it's unlikely!). The only time you want to avoid trace THC just to be on the safe side is if you are an athlete or a person who has regular drug testing for THC, or if you are in a country where no THC is allowable in non-prescription CBD products. If that is you, stick to 'THC-free broad-spectrum' CBD products and make sure the COA verifies this claim. For medical cannabis products, the THC percentage should also be listed along with the number of mg of THC per bottle/ml/capsule, depending on the form of the product. The THC dose is calculated in the same way as the CBD dose above.

Minor cannabinoids

If a product is full-spectrum or broad-spectrum, it means it also contains at least some minor cannabinoids in trace amounts alongside CBD if it is a hemp CBD wellness product (and alongside CBD and THC if it is a medical cannabis product), such as: THCA, CBDA, CBDV, CBN, CBC and CBG vs CBD isolate contains none of these.

Terpenes

Terpenes are often not reported on lab results, since HPLC is not very good at measuring them. Even when they are measured, it's often hard to give an exact amount, so they will just be reported as 'rich in X or Y terpene'. Another technique called gas chromatography/mass spectrometry (GC/MS) is a better way to measure terpenes, but not normally done on large batches so most products will not have a detailed report for terpenes outside a research setting currently.

Contaminants, solvent residue and heavy metals

The lab should also test for and report pesticide residue, solvent residue, heavy metals and other chemicals, such as synthetic cannabinoids like 'spice', which may be toxic to some organs and should not be consumed by humans (it is *not* botanical cannabis).

Microbiology testing

This looks for moulds and other microbes such as potentially harmful bacteria. Harmful moulds are not visible to the naked eye like they are in food, but they can be unsafe to inhale or ingest, and can grow on the cannabis if the conditions are too wet. Some moulds can also produce a poison, such as the aflatoxin made by some aspergillus mould strains, which can be a carcinogen and liver toxin in humans. Pathogenic bacteria that have been found on cannabis include strains of E. coli and staphylococcus, so again this is why testing for these things is so important, to ensure you are getting a safe, non-toxic product.

Where to find the COA for a product

Many websites will have the COA lab reports for their products listed online or as downloadable PDFs, or you can request them via email in some cases. Some very local, independent products may not have a COA, so if you want to use one of those products, I generally recommend sending a sample (or getting the seller to do so) to a certified third-party testing lab first to ensure it is safe.

Out-of-date lab reports

If a product was tested when it was produced but is then stored for a long time, or exposed to moisture (flower cannabis) or light (from being stored in a clear bottle instead of a dark amber one), it may have lost many of its active ingredients. The terpenes will be lost first, followed by some of the cannabinoids, which can be degraded by UV light. If the flowers have been stored without moisture-control packs, they could have developed mould even if they were mould-free when they were packaged at the growing and processing facility.

For additional information, see references[12, 13, 14, 15, 16, 17, 18, 19, 20, 21].

CHAPTER SIX

SO, IS IT SAFE?

Before trying any new cannabis or CBD product, I must advise you to speak to your doctor or healthcare professional to find out what is right for you, especially considering the official advice from multiple regulatory bodies on CBD at the time of writing, since a book can only ever be an educational tool, and should not be considered a replacement for your doctor's advice. However, to my knowledge at the time of writing, the only health problems (which have been increased liver enzymes or liver problems) from CBD have been in mice given 2460 mg/kg of body weight of CBD[1] and in a few cases of children treated with high dose (1000 mg) of purified CBD alongside other seizure medications (from the Epidiolex drug studies in epilepsy) which can also cause liver problems on their own even without CBD. This is very different for the low CBD doses used by most people for wellness and even most of my patients for more serious medical reasons. I have never had a serious adverse event from CBD in any patient or client who has used it. In other human studies on CBD, which is more applicable than in animals, doses of 600 mg and even 1500 mg doses have been well-tolerated. So in summary, even though we don't know everything yet, CBD and even medical cannabis with THC when used appropriately have a low risk of toxicity[2] and are safer than many over-the-counter medications and other herbal remedies many people take without a second thought. I believe because CBD is from the cannabis plant with a huge history of stigma surrounding its use, it has been approached more cautiously by regulatory and safety authorities than another supplement from a different plant would have been. As we get bigger data sets on CBD, I believe the safety issues around CBD in the doses used by most people will be put to bed and reflect what has been my personal and clinical experience.

Because cannabis is both a drug and a botanical medicine, it is easy to make the mistake of thinking that it is 100% safe since it's 'natural'. But as I point out to my patients and clients, just because something is natural does not mean it has zero risks. There are many toxic botanicals that can cause serious harm, or even kill you, even though they come from a plant and are totally natural.

Hemp CBD wellness products

CBD is generally a non-toxic substance in both humans and animals. There are very few true contraindications to trying it, especially at low doses, although there are a few caution areas, as with any substance that has a biological effect on our bodies so always check with your doctor.

In the UK, CBD wellness products (i.e. all CBD from hemp containing less than 0.2% THC) are classified as health and wellness supplements or 'food supplements' if they are ingested in the body (i.e. CBD oils, tinctures, sprays, gummies, edibles, drinks, etc.). They are not made as a medication or intended for medical use, unlike medical cannabis available by prescription. That being said, CBD does of course have medicinal qualities and its effects vary between individuals, by product and dosage used and for what purpose. Higher doses of CBD are normally used when the product is for medical use. CBD appears safe and non-toxic in humans in preliminary studies so far even at doses of up to 1500 mg/day[3] (to give you some context, the average non-prescription hemp CBD wellness product daily total dose is between 30 and 60 mg/day).

Like most herbal supplements, CBD may affect certain medications, and there are at least a few drug/herb interactions where caution is needed. Most significant interactions with CBD occur at doses much higher than 100 mg/day, according to the evidence we have so far, so CBD wellness products under this amount are likely low risk, but it's best to be cautious. In my clinical experience, I have never seen an issue occur between other wellness supplements and CBD so far. Another reason to check with your doctor is that CBD can affect your immune system and drugs that affect your immune response.

- History of heart problems, angina, irregular heartbeat, heart arrhythmia. In general you may still be able to use CBD, but under medical guidance. CBD may even benefit people with heart problems, according to preliminary research, but to be safe, always check with your doctor before starting anything.
- History of stroke or TIA.
- History of genetic blood-clotting disorders.
- History of any immune system disorder, if you are taking immunotherapy drugs or if you have a compromised immune system such as in cancer patients, HIV/AIDS or genetic immune deficiency disorders.
- If you are taking drugs such as blood thinners, or any heart medications.
- If you are taking anti-rejection drugs after having an organ transplant.[4]
- If you taking anti-seizure drugs (i.e. anti-epileptics), especially one called clobazam.
- If you are on immunotherapy drugs to treat cancer, since CBD may alter (decrease) the immune system's response to the drug therapy.

Although the side effects of low-dose wellness CBD products are virtually nil for most people, some people who are sensitive to supplements or medications may have mild and usually temporary side effects, which can include:

- Dizziness and mild low blood pressure. CBD is a mild vasorelaxant, meaning it can relax or make the blood vessels wider. This lowers blood pressure in the body, and may cause a dip in blood pressure by a few points. This mild decrease may cause people who already have low or borderline-low blood pressure to feel dizziness, particularly if they go quickly from sitting/lying to standing, or if they have been diagnosed with a condition like POTS, which is a collection of symptoms including low blood pressure, fainting or near-fainting episodes and racing heartbeat that can be accompanied by persistent fatigue. If this low blood effect occurs, generally just decreasing the dose and building it up again more slowly as tolerated is enough to overcome it.

- Drowsiness. Some people report a slight increase in drowsiness after taking CBD, although technically it is not a true side effect. This usually occurs at a single dose of 30 mg or more and is very rarely an issue. CBD in a pure form generally does not cause drowsiness. A drowsy reaction may be due to the strain of hemp being rich in myrcene terpenes, which can cause relaxation and drowsiness. Changing brands to one with less myrcene may help this symptom go away completely. Alternatively, if you are very stressed and wired due to high stress hormone and cortisol levels, you may experience unfamiliar tiredness as a result of the calming effect of CBD in the nervous system and stress system. In this case, your body is telling you to slow down and start reducing your stress load.

Given the above caveats, CBD products from hemp appear to so far have a good safety profile, especially at the average wellness doses of well under 100 mg/day, as long as they are actually CBD and not contaminated with THC, chemicals or other toxins. Many natural supplements and botanical medicines, especially those originating from certain countries (traditionally products made in China and India have had lots of issues), have been found to contain heavy metals like mercury and lead when sent to an independent lab for analysis. CBD is no different, especially since cannabis and hemp varieties suck up contaminants from the soil if they are grown in poor conditions. For this reason only products tested by a third-party laboratory and with a COA (certificate of analysis) report should be used (see the previous chapter). Many products on the shelves may be of questionable quality. The regulations in the UK for CBD wellness products are still quite lax, so quality is widely variable, although this is already starting to improve as the hemp and CBD industry evolves and regulations catch up.

Medical cannabis containing THC

As a group, cannabinoids are both non-toxic to organs and non-lethal in overdose, unlike drugs such as opioids and even some over-the- counter drugs that can damage organs in large amounts. That being said, cannabis containing THC above the trace amounts found in CBD hemp products may not be appropriate for everyone, just as alcohol is not appropriate for many people despite the fact that consuming large quantities of it is completely legal.

Compared to many of the prescription and even non-prescription drugs people routinely use, cannabis has less potential for side effects, as well as being non-toxic for most healthy people. This is especially the case in low doses and when used under the guidance of a doctor who understands cannabis. Some people at increased risk should not use THC-containing products unless under close supervision of a doctor specialising in this area, as the risks may be outweighed by any potential benefits.

Examples of where THC should generally be avoided include mental health conditions such as psychosis, schizophrenia and mania. That being said, very intriguing preliminary research on the relationship between THC and schizophrenia is showing us that in some cases, cannabis may help decrease the side effects from drugs needed to control the condition, and that a small amount of cannabis may even alleviate (but not cure) some symptoms alongside drug therapy, but it is still too early to say what this will mean for patients who suffer from these illnesses in terms of medical cannabis safety and use. For now, it is probably safest to avoid it completely in these cases, especially for the purposes of general advice.

Like most things in medicine, no rule is absolute for all patients and we are constantly learning more about cannabis and its medical uses. THC may slightly increase the risk of heart issues, especially in those who are higher risk already for things like heart attacks or strokes, which is why a doctor should always be consulted if any of these conditions apply to you:

- Psychosis (self or first-degree relative, i.e. a parent, sibling or child), including schizophrenia and schizoaffective disorders, as well as other causes of psychosis.
- Mania or bipolar disorder.
- Cannabis use disorder or cannabis addiction.
- Pregnancy and breastfeeding.
- Unstable cardiovascular (heart) disease.
- Recent heart attack.
- Any cardiac arrhythmia, including:
    - atrial fibrillation (avoid unless stable and rate-controlled and used under strict medical guidance by a heart specialist)
    - long QT syndrome (a disorder of the heart's electrical activity)
    - undiagnosed heart palpitations possibly related to a heart condition.**
- On anticoagulants (blood thinners) such as warfarin, due to the possible CBD interaction. In some cases they can be used together, but only under strict medical supervision with monitoring blood tests for blood clotting factors (in one case report, the blood clotting marker called the INR changed with CBD).[5]
- On cancer immunotherapy drugs, due to possible reduced response to the drug when mixed with cannabis (so far we think this is more to do with the CBD content vs the THC content). Consider when benefits may outweigh risks, such as in palliative care.
- Liver cirrhosis (advanced liver disease), especially if it is hepatitis C related, due to a possible effect of THC progressing the disease faster to liver fibrosis, although data is still inconclusive and some experts feel it poses minimal risk.[6, 7]

** For any cardiac issue patients, a heart specialist (cardiologist) doctor should be involved to ensure the heart issue is stable and to monitor the patient for THC-related side effects. I recommend very low-THC, high-CBD cannabis for these patients in a few cases, but the decision should be made on a case-by-case basis under medical supervision.

- On clobazam or other seizure/anti-epileptic drugs, especially if taking medical cannabis that contains doses of CBD >100 mg/day (you can use them together but only under strict medical supervision and monitoring blood levels of the drug to ensure it is in the safe range, since CBD may increase the drug level slightly).
- If you have a safety-sensitive job including operating machinery or driving (for THC products for daytime use).

I have found that most of my patients who only use high-CBD, low-THC medical cannabis products rarely experience any significant or lasting side effects under the dosage guidelines I recommend for them. When they do, these effects are mild and go away in a few weeks after tolerance develops, even with products higher in THC where this may be needed. For example, if we are trying to use medical cannabis to reduce high amounts of morphine and other opioid painkillers, THC is usually far less impairing or intoxicating than the opioids themselves. This is something patients tell me again and again: that they feel far more lucid even with higher-THC medical cannabis than they did on morphine or fentanyl.

That being said, a small number of people will be very sensitive to even low amounts of THC, especially if they have never taken it before. That is why using the 'start low, go slow' approach, and working with a doctor, is important in minimising the risk of any side effects of THC in medical cannabis.

Most common side effects of THC-containing cannabis

The most common side effects of THC-containing cannabis are usually mild and short-lived, although they can be scary if you don't expect them. I have had many a call from panicked family members, friends and patients themselves who have accidentally misdosed their cannabis oil and ended up overmedicated – aka high as a kite. I found this happened especially after Canada legalised cannabis, when customers bought over-the-counter high-THC cannabis from

a legal shop without a prescription. These products are sold officially for recreational use, but many people buy them intending to use
them medically or for a health reason, not because they want to get
stoned. The typical staff at these shops are often well-meaning but
medically untrained salespeople, not doctors. Although it may sound
funny, it can be very discombobulating, especially if you have never
had prior experience with drugs, or suffer with anxiety, or hate feeling
out of control.

These potential THC side effects are also dose-dependent –
meaning that they are not common at micro doses under 10 mg and
very rare at doses under 5 mg. However, if you accidentally took, say,
70 mg of THC, especially if you were unused to it, you might be in for
an interesting few hours to say the least. In the most severe scenario,
some chocolate bars with cannabis sold in US states where recreational cannabis is legal contain enough THC (100–200 mg!) to trigger
a heart attack in someone who is already at high risk if they ate it all at
once. These are not doses I would recommend for anyone, and certainly the doses I use medically are way below that (normally between
5 and 20 mg/day).

If they do occur, the most common THC side effects are:

- increased heart rate
- racing heartbeat
- heart palpitations
- feeling out of control or panicked
- dizziness
- dry mouth
- increased appetite
- fatigue or grogginess
- paranoia/dysphoria (rare)
- anxiety/panic
- impaired co-ordination

Potential long-term effects of THC

There are some studies that show chronic daily THC use may impair short-term memory and disrupt concentration in some people. It is worth keeping in mind that these studies were done on high-THC, low-CBD smoked recreational cannabis rather than medical cannabis. These effects, including effects on the brain that can be seen on brain imaging studies, reverse themselves within three months of stopping THC, so that is quite reassuring based on what we know so far.

For example, one of the brain changes seen with daily chronic THC use is a reduced density of CB1 receptors, but this effect returns to baseline within 28 days in most brain regions except the hippocampus, which also recovers but more slowly. Taking CBD alongside THC may be protective against this effect, although more research is needed to confirm these case findings. Basically what that means in plain English is that the brain adapts to having lots of THC hanging around and takes down some receptor sites for THC and endocannabinoids, since there are lots floating around. This happens with many drugs taken for chronic conditions and is a way in which the brain and body try to constantly regulate themselves. The important thing is that once cannabis with THC is stopped, the brain returns to pre-cannabis receptor levels and does not lose its ability to self-regulate back to baseline.

Cannabis 'discontinuation' syndrome

This is the term for symptoms of stopping THC-containing cannabis 'cold turkey', and does not apply to hemp CBD products. Symptoms may include: insomnia, irritability, anxiety, appetite changes and nausea. This can happen with my medical cannabis patients who go on an overseas trip where they cannot take their cannabis (they might be using a THC oil to help with sleep or a daytime THC product for pain or other medical symptoms on a daily basis). In order to prevent this, I tell them to inform my office well in advance of trips outside of

Canada so we can meet and discuss options and, if needed, wean them off gradually before their trip if they are travelling somewhere they cannot see a doctor to get medical cannabis legally. I once had a lovely elderly patient ask me if he could bring his medical cannabis to Saudi Arabia to visit his family there, and of course that was definitely not possible, so we had to wean him slowly down off it before his trip. He did tell me that some people in the Middle East do smoke (illegal) hashish for medical reasons, but behind closed doors. I advised him (obviously!) that it was best to avoid any black market cannabis on his trip due to the very strict legal penalties in that part of the world regarding cannabis of any sort.

Cannabis discontinuation syndrome is normally mild, self-limiting, not dangerous and lasts for less than two weeks (usually around seven days or less in most people). For medical cannabis, which tends to contain CBD as well as THC, this syndrome is usually very mild. For someone smoking high-THC recreational cannabis with nearly no CBD, stopping abruptly without tapering down the dose may have more severe symptoms, which, although not dangerous, can be uncomfortable in the short term. The biggest issue with cannabis discontinuation in medical cannabis patients is the lack of pain relief/symptom control when they cannot have their cannabis; they may have to go back on other drugs for their trip to help them manage symptoms until they can resume their cannabis therapy.

High-THC smoked cannabis in adolescent brains

It does seem that chronic smoked cannabis use before the brain is fully matured (in teens and adolescents) may change the brain more in areas of decision-making and memory and may lead to long-term effects, at least in some people. Use after the age of 25 appears not to have this long-term association after people stop smoking cannabis. This is why I strongly discourage recreational cannabis use in teens and young adults, especially high-THC, low-CBD cannabis. Medical cannabis in these age groups, however, is sometimes still appropriate but should be taken only under medical guidance after careful assessment by a doctor and weighing the possible benefits and other alternatives against the risks. If it is used, lower-THC, high-CBD cannabis should be tried first, usually in a longer-acting form like an oil or capsule.

THC and fertility

Another area of caution when it comes to taking THC is with women and men of reproductive age, due to possible fertility effects. A definite risk to fertility has not been proven in women, although THC may affect the menstrual cycle in some women. Some preliminary studies have shown in men that THC may cause reduced sperm counts and motility (see Chapters Thirteen and Fourteen for more details). It is probable that these effects are dose-dependent and more likely with chronic heavy daily use.

What to do if you accidentally take too much THC

In general, accidental overmedication with THC is not life-threatening, unless you have an unstable heart problem (in which case, see below). In most cases, the feelings may be uncomfortable, but they are manageable at home. If you are feeling intoxicated, panicky or out of control, put on some calming music, get yourself in a safe space, either lying down in bed or on a couch, and start practising slow, gentle breathing. I have a technique called 'tissue box breathing' (sometimes called 'the healing breath'), which I regularly practise with patients who suffer with anxiety and stress. I get them to lie down on the exam table and I put a tissue box on their stomach, on top of the belly button. As they breathe in, the tissue box will move upwards. As they exhale through the mouth with a gentle 'haaaaaaa' sound, they can watch the tissue box move back down. It sounds almost ridiculously simple, but the effect is instantly calming for the nervous system, and helps regain a sense of control in the mind and body.

If you are feeling intoxicated, you should, of course, avoid driving, using machinery or going to work; just wait it out. If you have over-medicated with a vaporised cannabis product, the worst is usually over in less than an hour and the effects usually wear off completely in two to three hours. If you ate a cannabis edible or took an oral oil, the results can last longer – around six hours or so. In this situation, prepare a 'nest' at home with comfy clothes, blankets, some herbal tea, calming music and a few movies to keep you entertained and comfortable while the effects wear off. I should add that this level of discomfort after taking medical cannabis is very rare – I am extremely specific about dosing with my patients, so that even if they make a slight mistake, it is rarely enough to cause more than a mild sense of intoxication, but if you've really overdone it, this is the best strategy. I also recommend calling a friend, partner or loved one you can rely on and letting them know how you are feeling so they can keep an eye on you if needed.

However, if you ever experience what you think may be chest pain or shortness of breath after taking THC, always call 999 to get immediate emergency medical attention. In a healthy person without heart issues, the chest tightness and shortness of breath that can happen after taking too much THC is generally due to a mild panic attack rather than a heart attack, but because the symptoms are almost impossible to tell apart on your own, you need to get checked out immediately. If you already have a heart issue, or think you might, it is even more important to get to hospital as soon as possible. Never be embarrassed about getting checked out by a doctor – this is something I emphasise to all of my patients. If something doesn't feel right, seek medical attention straight away, just like you would with any other potentially serious medication reaction.

> Sometimes it's hard to judge if you are feeling intoxicated, or if you may be impaired for activities like driving. Download an app onto your phone such as DRUID, which measures your potential level of impairment for driving by putting you through a series of simple performance tasks to measure balance and reaction time. Also follow the precautionary principle: if you have any doubts at all about whether you are impaired, stay safe and just don't drive. This is the same precaution you should take with any other medication, including over-the-counter allergy pills that can make you drowsy, or other prescription medications.

Is euphoria a side effect?

In medical school, the only thing we learned about cannabis was that it could make people psychotic, and that a side effect of it was euphoria, which in plain English means joy or happiness. I could never figure out (and no one could ever explain to me) exactly why euphoria was such a bad thing – for example, if you have even mild depression, a bit of euphoria is probably quite nice! That being said, if the euphoria happens and you have a condition like bipolar depression and it tips you over into mania, that is not desirable (which is why high THC should be avoided by those who are bipolar).

It struck me that this general labelling of euphoria as something to be feared may also be a product of one of the weaknesses of the modern Western medicine system. In its sterilised, rational and reductionist approach to the human body, it can fail to recognise the importance of joy, connection, human experience and the creation of 'peak experiences' that often make life feel worth living and which bind us together as humans. I also think it is probably true that most medical doctors may have had little experience with cannabis and other substances such as psychedelics like psilocybin (from 'magic mushrooms'), and things we have not experienced or that we do not understand we often fear as a default. We now know, for example, that psilocybin, much like cannabis, has therapeutic potential. In the US, it has just been granted FDA approval for 'breakthrough drug status' for use in depression, while in the UK, multiple major studies are under way at some of the top universities looking at how such natural compounds may be used medically to treat treatment-resistant depression and other mental health conditions where modern drugs have failed.

> ## DO CANNABIS AND ALCOHOL MIX?
>
> THC will enhance the effects of alcohol, and vice versa, which is why combining THC with even a single glass of wine may lead to stronger feelings of impairment and intoxication than either on their own. The reaction has a huge individual variation from person to person, due to the breakdown enzymes in the liver being unique to each of us. The bottom line is, if you are new to cannabis and still finding your steady-state dose, or changing products, it's best to avoid taking it with alcohol until things are stabilised. Then you can try introducing a single unit of alcohol with a meal (to slow absorption) and see how it makes you feel, ensuring that you do not have to drive or operate machinery afterwards. I recommend that if you are going to mix them, experiment at home on a weekend just in case you do feel impaired. A cannabis dose that would not normally cause impairment may impair you when combined with a glass of wine or other alcoholic drink. That being said, once things are stable, many of my patients who take medical cannabis do enjoy the occasional glass of wine with a meal.

Cannabis addiction and problem cannabis use

Cannabis and THC do not carry a risk of physical dependency like drugs such as morphine and other opioids. However, chronic high-THC, low-CBD cannabis use, especially unsupervised recreational use, can lead to a cannabis use disorder or cannabis addiction in around

9% of regular cannabis users, based on the current data.[8] Addiction means the development of a mental dependency, including cravings, as well as increased use despite negative life consequences. I should reiterate that these figures and statistics refer to unsupervised recreational use, and not to medical cannabis users, where addiction is very rare when used under proper guidance. Developing an addiction to medical cannabis is a problem I have never encountered after treating thousands of patients.

Factors like age and sex may affect how cannabis interacts with our own endocannabinoid system, something that is being investigated by Dr Lili Galindo at Cambridge University in order to understand who may be at higher risk of adverse mental effects from THC-containing cannabis.

I believe it is good to be aware of any potential addiction risks, especially if you have a history of addiction to other substances. If you experience two or more of the following signs and symptoms, you may be at risk of or experiencing a cannabis dependency:

* Excessive daily use of cannabis beyond the amount needed to control medical symptoms.
* Needing higher and higher doses of cannabis and THC beyond this amount.
* Compulsion or cravings to use cannabis whenever available, not just related to medical use.

If you are concerned you may be at risk, even if you do not meet these criteria, talk to your medical doctor asap!

The risk to lungs of inhaled cannabis

With smoked cannabis there is a risk of lung irritation from heavy chronic use, due to the burning of the plant material. This in turn may increase the risk of chronic obstructive pulmonary disease (COPD) in some individuals, though the research is not clear. The question of whether smoked cannabis may cause lung cancer is also still unclear.

It is known that cannabis smoke does contain some cancer-causing chemicals called hydrocarbons (e.g. benzopyrene, which is also in cigarette smoke), though unlike tobacco smoke, which has only bad stuff that can cause cancers, cannabis smoke contains some anti-cancer and anti-inflammatory chemicals too, which counteract (at least to some degree) the nasty bits. However, especially with medical cannabis patients (who 9 times out of 10 have an inflammatory component to at least one of their ailments), smoking anything can add fuel to the inflammation fire, and avoiding smoking altogether is the best way to reduce any potential harm to the lungs.

These risks of burning the cannabis flower material can be mostly avoided by vaporising it at a temperature setting below 217°C. The cannabinoids CBC and THCV are the last two to vaporise off, at 220°C, so you may miss these chemicals in the vapour, but it's probably worth that to avoid getting the bad stuff boiling off, such as toxic naphthalene. Big studies are still lacking, so I tend to take the most cautious approach based on the science that we do know so far.

In order for dried herb vaporisers to be ready and safe for use with cannabis, they need to be heated first without any flower in them to burn off any potential chemical residues from the manufacturing process. A good-quality vaporiser will come with exact instructions on how to do this, and there are also many YouTube video tutorials on how to clean a cannabis dried herbal vaporiser prior to first use (see also Chapter Five). If you already have COPD or another lung disease, such as recurrent bronchitis or fibrosis, using other methods besides inhaling cannabis may be best for you, and this is generally what I recommend for such cases. However, some types of severe pain with spasms that come on suddenly respond best to inhaled cannabis, so if someone only has mild COPD or asthma, we weigh up the options of adding vaporised cannabis. In these cases, the bronchodilatory (opening the airway) effect of THC can often alleviate an asthma or COPD acute attack temporarily, similar to a Ventolin puffer (although it is not standard treatment for this indication).

Can THC cause a heart attack, stroke or palpitations?

THC can increase the workload on the heart, which can be danger-ous for those with weak hearts or arrhythmias, as it can strain it to the point where it can't keep up. In large doses, THC can also increase the stress and anxiety response, especially in those unused to it, which again can cause more strain on the heart's pumping action. If you were to take a huge dose of THC and were already at high risk of having a heart attack or a stroke, or had pre-existing heart or blood vessel disease, the THC could trigger a life-threatening arrhythmia, heart attack or stroke. In extremely rare cases it could even cause death if it triggered a massive heart attack and medical attention was not received in time.

The only case reports I have heard of a fatal heart attack caused by a huge dose of THC were in unsupervised non-medical use of rec-reational cannabis. I have never heard of a case of medical cannabis causing death when used under medical supervision, and no cases have been reported in the published research as far as I am aware. The research on the association between cannabis use and cardiac problems is from smoked recreational cannabis with higher THC, not medical cannabis, which is usually lower in THC and higher in CBD and monitored by a doctor like any other medication. That being said, I have turned down patients for THC-containing medical canna-bis who have had an unstable heart condition. It's not always a happy conversation, but it is my duty to 'do no harm' first.

For additional information, see references[9, 10, 11, 12, 13].

Todd's story: the mystery arrhythmia trigger

Todd, a man in his mid-fifties, came to see me for medical cannabis for chronic pain. He was not new to medical cannabis and had already been prescribed it by another doctor, who did not actually know much about botanical medicine or cannabis and so essentially gave him a blank pre-scription so he could experiment and see what he liked best. He was not monitoring the use closely, which became clear when we chatted.

It turned out Todd was smoking a high-THC strain of cannabis, not vaporising it or using oral products higher in CBD as I would have recommended. This was a concern because he suffered with a heart rhythm problem called atrial fibrillation (A-fib), which can be made worse or triggered by THC. When I saw Todd initially and quizzed him about his medication history, it became clear that his A-fib symptoms were intensifying after starting the high-THC cannabis. A recent acute episode, which resulted in an emergency hospital visit, matched up with a large amount of high-THC cannabis smoked that day and the day before in an attempt to curb a pain flare-up. The previous doctor had not given him any specific instructions on what types of medical cannabis he should be using.

I told him that I thought it likely the high-THC strain he had chosen, although it helped his pain, was probably contributing to more flare-ups of his heart condition. After some initial convincing, he agreed to stop smoking cannabis completely and change to vaporising and oils by mouth. We put him on a medical cannabis oil with a higher CBD and lower THC ratio (around 5:1) as his base. He still needed some THC because his back pain was very severe, and before medical cannabis he had been dependent on opioids for pain control. For acute breakthrough pain, we added a vaporised balanced strain, with slightly more CBD than THC (2:1) but with enough THC to still help him acute episodes quickly. That meant we cut his THC content in half instantly.

Adding a CBD-rich oil product with enough THC to give him a background of longer-acting pain relief helped Todd to get ahead of the pain and inflammation so he had fewer acute flare-ups. Changing from smoking to using the vaporiser reduced the risks to his lungs and any inflammatory by-products that could affect the cardiovascular system negatively. After all these changes, Todd's heart condition became stable, he had no more hospital trips for palpitations, his pain was eased and he felt better overall and less groggy.

Todd's story is a strong example of why, for anyone with heart problems, close monitoring by a doctor is essential to ensure the treatment is safe and effective.

Drug/herb interactions

Like everything we ingest, from food additives to drugs and herbs, cannabis and cannabinoids from the plant get broken down in our liver by special enzymes. So it is possible for drug/herb interactions to occur with medical cannabis and CBD. There are not many clinically significant interactions between cannabis and most other drugs that have so far been proven, but it is always best to be cautious, just as you would be when adding any new medication, even the birth control pill or an over-the-counter drug.

THC and CBD are the most studied of the cannabinoids in terms of their metabolism in the liver. The enzymes that break them down are the same ones that break down many other drugs and herbs. Exploring all of the numerous complex drug/herb interaction possibilities involving the liver's enzyme system (called the cytochrome P450 system) is beyond the scope of this book, but it is safe to say that the effect that cannabis, especially at high doses, may have on other drugs is unquantifiable. This basically means it's unknown due to the lack of published studies on the thousands of different drug/cannabis combinations. That may sound pretty scary, but the fact is that most drugs suffer from the same issue. The research in drug/herb and drug/drug interactions is focused mainly on a select number of higher-risk drugs that can interact with each other, causing decreased or increased blood levels that can be significant if that drug has a narrow therapeutic index (safe level). Cannabis in general has a wide therapeutic index, thankfully, and only a few drugs have published evidence about how they interact with CBD and/or THC.

These are the key drug/herb interactions to be aware of:

- Warfarin. THC and CBD can increase warfarin levels.[14]
- Alcohol. May increase THC levels when the two are taken together.[15, 16]
- Theophylline (a drug used for COPD/chronic lung disease, although not as common now as 10 years ago). Smoked cannabis can decrease theophylline levels.[17]

- Clobazam. In children treated with CBD for epilepsy, CBD increased clobazam levels.[18]
- Immunotherapy agents for non-small-cell lung cancer, renal cancer and melanoma. Retrospective observational study from Israel showed decreased response to drug but no difference in progression-free survival or overall survival.[19]
- Tacrolimus. An anti-organ-rejection and immunotherapy drug. May have an interaction with CBD at very high doses (over 1000 mg of CBD in the study published).
- Other anti-organ rejection drugs such as Cellcept. No published evidence, but similar drug type to tacrolimus.
- Tamoxifen. Unpublished data collection ongoing from a colleague in Canada doing clinical trials. It remains unknown whether THC decreases response.
- St John's wort. No published studies of specific interaction with cannabis, THC or CBD, but St John's wort is one of the best-known herbal supplements for drug/herb interactions due to its ability to induce (increase activity in) enzymes and alter many different drug levels, so I generally do not use it with cannabis, especially if the patient is on many other medications.

There are no published reports of any problematic interactions between cannabis and other botanical medicines. That being said, I would generally avoid combining high-THC and kava due to their combined sedative effects. Generally, the other botanicals and natural supplements discussed in this book are ones I have used without issue alongside cannabis medicines with thousands of my patients, using a 'start low, go slow' approach and adding one thing at a time in most cases.

Safe storage away from kids and pets

As with all medications and botanical medicines, it is important to avoid accidental ingestion of cannabis by kids or pets. In children with certain conditions, such as treatment-resistant seizure disorders or other severe developmental disorders, cannabis may be very helpful in a controlled medical environment under the care of a paediatrician who understands cannabis and CBD. However, it is not recommended for healthy children.

THC can make pets very disoriented due to the effect on the brain's balance centres in animals, which are more sensitive even than human brains in this respect, so it's important (especially if you have a Labrador, aka garbage disposal unit!) to keep cannabis out of reach. CBD oil from hemp, on the other hand, without measurable THC, can help calm anxious pets and appears safe, but always consult your vet first if you want to give it a try. Many of my patients have given their pets CBD after having great results themselves, and I have seen it help their dogs (and a few cats) with arthritis pain, separation anxiety and hyperactivity. Hemp seed oil is also a healthy oil that may help their coats. More and more pet CBD products are emerging in the US and Canada, although currently CBD is not legal as a pet medicine or food ingredient in the UK (despite the fact that it's legal for humans – something I find quite funny!).

To ensure everyone's safety, keep your cannabis products in a lockbox to which only you have the combination or key. I advise purchasing a box big enough to hold moisture-control packs for your cannabis flower, if you use that, as well as all other products. UV light (e.g. from sunlight) will degrade your CBD and medical cannabis products, so the box should be opaque as well.

Positive side effects of cannabis and CBD

Although there are some areas of caution when it comes to THC-containing cannabis, there are very few situations in which CBD hemp products or high-CBD, very low-THC medical cannabis products cannot be tried. I always feel it's important to point out the positive side effects of cannabis medicine therapy that I have witnessed first-hand with the thousands of patients I have seen:

- Increased uptake of mindfulness and meditation. In many studies, including a Harvard study on mindfulness meditation, people must stick with the practice daily for 8 weeks or so to start seeing a sustained benefit. When people can use CBD or medical cannabis as a tool to help wind down their mind enough to engage in meditation or other relaxation practices, they are able to stick with these practices long enough to see a benefit for mental health and stress levels. Pre-cannabis or CBD, sticking to a practice for more than a few days was impossible for most of my patients who suffered with chronic pain, toxic stress levels and/or anxiety, due to an inability to calm their systems down for long enough each day and sit through the discomfort of learning the techniques.

- An enhanced doctor–physician relationship. Many of my patients felt completely failed by the medical system before coming to see me for medical cannabis. Through working together using cannabis, they have regained their trust in doctors and are able to partner with their care teams to improve their health outcomes.

- A sense of internal control and hope. When faced with a severe chronic illness where the disease itself may be incurable, quality of life is the goal. Because cannabis often works so well for symptoms that were previously uncontrollable, it provides respite from suffering and helps patients regain a sense of control over their symptoms and their life. This is something that has often been taken away from them due to their illness experience.

- Reduced pill burden. Cannabis often dramatically reduces the number of prescription and over-the-counter medications people require on a daily basis to cope with symptoms such as pain, inflammation, anxiety, poor sleep, stress and fatigue. In the best cases this has included completely coming off painkillers, opioids, benzodiazepines, sleeping pills and other high-side-effect drugs.

- Weight loss. Many of my patients lose weight after starting medical cannabis, contrary to the belief that cannabis munchies will make people gain weight. Using high-CBD strains seems to have the potential to improve blood sugar control, a finding that is starting to be supported by preliminary research into the positive metabolic effects of CBD and other cannabinoids in pre-diabetes, diabetes and metabolic syndrome.

- Increased exercise. When people are experiencing less pain and lower inflammation, they have more energy and are able to start and maintain a regular exercise programme.
- Return to work. Contrary to the notion that cannabis makes people lazy, many of my patients on disability have been able to resume work in some form, either part- or full-time.
- Dramatically improved quality of life. Every week, one of my patients will say to me that cannabis has changed their life. They are often adamant that I write that down, because they feel so passionate about recording their experience and results within the medical community, especially after cannabis use was demonised for so many decades.

In summary, medical cannabis and CBD wellness products generally have a very good safety record, despite the last 100 years of being treated like a dangerous drug in most countries. Like any therapy, however, there are some risks, mainly from THC-containing products, for certain people and if certain drugs are also being taken, so always consult with your doctor first before starting cannabis products.

Part Two

CHAPTER SEVEN

IMPROVING BRAIN WELLNESS, BRAIN AGEING AND NEUROLOGICAL DISORDERS

Peak brain performance and neurodegenerative brain diseases like dementia may not appear to have much in common at first glance. However, optimal brain states and progressive neurological brain diseases are at opposite ends of the same brain health spectrum. And the more we discover about the brain and how it works, the more clear it seems that the same factors that keep our brains healthy and happy and high-functioning (like the ability to buffer inflammation and toxins, remove waste and keep all the brain chemicals balanced) are the same ones that can become dysfunctional and cause brain disease states. This dysfunction is seen at its most extreme in conditions like Alzheimer's, Parkinson's and other brain diseases that are part of a group of diseases doctors call neuropathological, which means a state of 'brain gone wrong'. These conditions are all slightly different, of course, but they share many similarities and all seem to involve endocannabinoid system dysfunction, which is why plant cannabinoids seem to help with so many of them.

Multiple sclerosis, which is included in this chapter, can be thought of as both a neurodegenerative disease and an autoimmune disease. It used be a mystery to scientists how it could be both, but we know now that the immune system and the brain and nervous system are intricately connected. Even the protein called beta-amyloid, thought initially to be the cause of Alzheimer's, is now thought to be an immune reaction gone wrong. Cannabinoids have an effect on both our brain and nervous systems via the good old endocannabinoid system.

In addition to my medical work with people who are ill, I also work at the other end of the spectrum, in the realm of peak brain performance. I have run peak performance programmes and resilience training, with clients ranging from Fortune 500 CEOs to professional athletes and actors, who take part in order to maximise their brain performance. We use a variety of tools, including EEG brain scanning (to help guide and customise the wellness plan based on brain signatures) and neurofeedback brain training, as well as diet, mind-body and lifestyle, and botanical medicines and supplements. CBD, in particular CBD from hemp (since it is more widely accessible to clients from many countries), has become a main feature in the 'supplement stack' we use, and clients continually rave about the difference they feel it has made to them. A few clients based in the US and Canada have also strategically added cannabis with micro-dosed THC into the mix, with beneficial effects.

So whether you are currently suffering with a neurodegenerative brain disease (or trying to help a loved one who is), or you just want to optimise your brain function for prevention and improve your brain ageing story, CBD and cannabis may have something to offer you.

My patients' special green juice recipe

In many small West Coast communities where I practise in BC, many of my patients live healthy, independent lives well into their late nineties and grow their own vegetables. Some of them also grew cannabis on their land, and instead of using it to get high, they would put the leaves through a juicer in the morning along with some spinach from the garden to make a very special but non-intoxicating green super juice that they swore kept them fit as a fiddle.

This was before I was prescribing cannabis medicines, but I became intrigued by this use and started to do some research as to what was in raw cannabis that might be beneficial for health. I discovered that by juicing the leaves and even the flower itself, my patients were actually getting THCA, the non-intoxicating precursor to THC. THCA seems to have a variety of health benefits with zero downsides – except that it requires a lot of juicing and a very high volume of material, which you could probably only reasonably afford if you grew a decent amount of your own cannabis outdoors. It is not exactly an efficient way to use it, but interesting nonetheless, and considering how healthy these people were into old age, who am I to argue with the results?

THC enhances brain performance and reverses brain ageing

A recent research study[1] looked at the brain and cognitive function of patients who were being treated with medical cannabis for chronic ailments. Their brain function was tested before starting medical cannabis, and then three months after, and results showed that their cognitive performance had improved. This improvement included brain performance and activation patterns in areas of the brain involved with executive function in the cingulate cortex and frontal lobes. The researchers concluded that instead of cannabis hurting brain function, these results were suggestive of a potential normalisation of brain function when it was not functioning optimally. They also found that the studied medical cannabis patients improved in multiple health-related measures and general well-being, as well as decreasing their use of potentially brain-harming and addictive medications such as opioids and benzodiazepines. (Note that this study was on medical cannabis and not on smoked recreational black market cannabis, which has not been shown to improve cognitive function.)

Another study in mice recently showed that cannabis can actually profoundly reverse brain ageing,[2] at least in senior-citizen mice, while a further study showed enhanced learning and memory and a change in brain structure and brain networks towards a more youthful brain age.[3]

In contrast to the beneficial effect on older adult brains, as previously explored, THC may have the opposite effect on healthy adolescent brains in teens and possibly into the early twenties, possibly disturbing a previously well-balanced endocannabinoid system. The only exception may be in teens with epilepsy and other neurological disorders, where the brain is not functioning normally; in these cases, CBD with a low dose of THC may actually help. The benefits in cases where medications have failed, and cannabis is prescribed by a paediatric specialist doctor under close supervision, may outweigh the risks.

If you don't currently have a brain disorder but are interested in healthy brain ageing and peak brain performance, preliminary evidence suggests that taking low doses of cannabinoids may be beneficial in later life. They may even help restore disrupted circadian rhythms in advanced ageing.[4] (Circadian rhythms are our daily physiologic patterns that control every aspect of brain and body function via the brain 'pacemaker' called the suprachiasmatic nucleus.)

A plant chemical approach to preventing and even reversing premature brain ageing

Some researchers have proposed taking a phytochemical (plant chemical) approach to helping fight diseases associated with brain ageing. Even though this may sound initially like a step back from using modern science, the most helpful conventional drugs used in Alzheimer's, the cholinesterase inhibitors, are compounds isolated from plants, such as a plant chemical called galantamine, found in the snowdrop. Research in cell and animal models suggests that cannabinoids as a group are important for neurogenesis, or new brain cell growth, in adult human brains, especially in certain areas like the hippocampus. While THC on its own in very high amounts may impair short-term memory temporarily, other cannabinoids may actually aid memory.[5]

We also know that terpenes (from cannabis and other plants) can cross the blood–brain barrier,[6] which means they can impact our brain directly. Terpenes, flavonoids and similar plant compounds may have neuroprotective effects that may prove beneficial in various neuropsychiatric and neurodegenerative disorders.

Numerous species of sage, and Spanish sage in particular, have been shown in multiple studies[7] to have cognitive enhancing effects and may be useful in these abnormal brain-ageing diseases. A recent study found that sage might help with prevention of such diseases, while another study found that it enhanced memory and attention in healthy older adults.[8, 9] Interestingly, the main plant chemicals responsible for these effects, monoterpenes, are also thought to be major bioactive chemicals in the cannabis plant, including one specific monoterpene called alpha-pinene,[10] which is known to enhance memory.

For my wellness clients who want to incorporate natural supplements and botanicals for brain performance and anti-ageing, I combine other botanicals with cannabis to give a natural brain boost, and also use them myself to help with focus, memory and general cognition support for the normal brain stresses of modern life.

CBD cocktails, anyone?

In addition to direct positive effects on brain ageing and neuroprotection, cannabis (and CBD in particular) may also be useful in promoting healthier habits, including helping us break some of the bad brain habits like overconsumption of alcohol. In a recent study, treatment with CBD helped to decrease cravings and reduce the amount of alcohol people drank, as well as protect their liver against some of the toxic effects of alcohol.[11] Recent years have seen the rise of CBD dinner parties and cannabis dinners in places like Canada, California and Colorado, New York and, even more recently, London. I have personally been to several CBD dinner parties where people drank minimally or not at all, and instead feasted on CBD-infused foods and drinks, much to my contentment, since I generally avoid alcohol for wellness reasons. At every one of these get-togethers, there were a few people who had never tried CBD or cannabis and who swore by the end of the night (after having no alcohol) that they felt more relaxed and generally better than normal after consuming in total over the evening around 60 mg of CBD per person.

CBD has the potential to change the way we socialise and the tools we use as social lubricants. More and more people are cutting down on their alcohol consumption or even choosing not to drink altogether as part of a wellness lifestyle. CBD and cannabis may replace alcohol as the go-to substance of choice for socialising in the near future, with almost no downsides (at least with hemp CBD and low-THC, high-CBD cannabis).

Artists and creatives have used cannabis for centuries to help assist with creativity and changing brain states, and the CBD movement has brought this into the mainstream with a super-safe alternative to black market cannabis.

How to use CBD wellness products (hemp CBD) for brain wellness

- Use a full-spectrum/broad-spectrum CBD oil.
- Look out for CBC – this minor cannabinoid has potent anti-inflammatory effects and may promote neurogenesis (new brain cells) in cell models.[12]
- Look for these beneficial terpenes:
  - alpha-pinene – may help with memory specifically
  - beta-caryophyllene – anti-inflammatory.

Starting dose and titrating up

For brain wellness, there is no standard dose. To make it cost-effective, you may want to start with between 5 mg and 10 mg of CBD 2–3 times a day with meals. If you also have another reason for trying CBD (such as chronic fatigue, burnout, anxiety, etc.), you may want to start with a higher dose and refer to the chapter relating to your specific issue for how to target it, or try a high tech product that is more absorbable, which means you would need less CBD to get the same result.

Remember: there is no specific perfect dose that works for everyone exactly the same way, because each person's endocannabinoid system and their balance is unique. So self-titration, starting low and slow with your dosing, is the name of the game as to how much CBD to add to your brain-wellness stack.

CBD may be most useful in terms of brain wellness and supporting brain performance when taken as part of what is called a nootropic stack. This is the term used in peak performance medicine for a supplement plan taken to to support brain performance, and can include natural supplements and botanicals.

The nootropic stack for brain wellness: non-cannabis helpers to consider

These botanicals have been used traditionally in some cases for thousands of years to help with brain function, cognition, mental sharpness and healthy ageing. More recent studies have revealed the very real beneficial effects they can have on the brain,[13] and because herbal medicine works by synergy, combining them may give a greater benefit than using a single herb on its own.

- Ginkgo biloba. A traditional Chinese medicine herb used for centuries for improving memory due to poor circulation (may improve vascular, or blood vessel, health within the brain and nervous system).
- Bacopa monnieri, or brahmi. A traditional Ayurvedic medicine herb used in India for centuries as a neuroprotectant and brain tonic to enhance memory and learning and help with stress and anxiety. It contains dozens of plant chemicals that contribute to this effect and is one of the most common herbals for older adults I encountered during my time in India. It is often used with other herbs like ashwagandha.
- Huperzine A. Extracted from Chinese club moss, this is a natural cholinesterase inhibitor, which mimics the effect of the most common pharmaceutical drug (donepezil) used to treat cognitive

impairment in dementia. According to some authors, it may equal or possibly even surpass the efficacy of the drug version, and with fewer side effects. Small preliminary studies have also shown it to be effective at enhancing cognition in Alzheimer's disease patients.[14, 15, 16]

- Curcumin with black pepper. Curcumin, from the turmeric plant, as well as whole root turmeric extract, is a neuroprotectant, an anti-inflammatory and may help with prevention of brain degenerative disorders. This is due to its ability to enhance brain-derived neurotrophic factor (BDNF), which stimulates the growth and survival of healthy neurons (brain cells).

A brain-support diet

In addition to taking botanical supplements, there are several dietary changes that can support the healthy functioning of the brain.

- Mediterranean diet; low-GI diet.[17, 18]
- Increase foods high in omega-3 fatty acids – fatty fish such as wild salmon, and small fish like anchovies and herring.
- Swap mixed vegetable oil for extra-virgin cold-pressed olive oil. Mixed, highly processed vegetable oil may be pro-inflammatory and lacks the good flavonoids and other plant chemicals in cold-pressed olive oil that contribute to brain and heart health.
- Eat a diet that is high in foods such as:
  - garlic and alliums (allicin) – high in sulphur, neuroprotective and help support detoxification in the liver
  - red grapes, red wine, tomatoes – these all contain resveratrol, which is a powerful antioxidant and neuroprotectant against toxins, stress and premature brain cell death
  - green tea – a source of epigallocatechin gallate, a powerful antioxidant and neuroprotectant against brain plaques like beta-amyloid, which are seen in brains with dementia; may decrease the risk of Parkinson's by 8% by drinking just one cup of green tea a day

- hot peppers – they contain capsaicin, which may help in brain cell-to-cell communication and antioxidant protection/neuroprotectant
- high-flavonoid foods such as apples, berries, dark chocolate and citrus fruits – flavonoids cross the blood–brain barrier and may aid in brain protection and anti-ageing effects[19]
- a wide variety of culinary spices and herbs – add as many herbs and spices as possible to your diet, as they are thought to contribute to the anti-inflammatory and antioxidant potential that is neuroprotective for the brain, and also help protect against environmental toxins, pollutants and stress-induced damage.

How to use medical cannabis products for brain wellness

Only try this under the supervision of a doctor and, of course, if medical cannabis (containing THC) is legal where you live.

- Start with a high-CBD cannabis oil as your base. This is best for minimising any THC-associated side effects while still providing low micro doses of THC that may also be neuroprotective along with CBD and the other plant chemicals.
- Average starting dose: 5 mg of CBD 2x/day using a high CBD, low-THC cannabis oil, which will give you a micro dose of THC if using a CBD to THC ratio of 20:1.
- You can stay at this micro dose if the main goal is using it as a supplement along with other nootropics in a stack; alternatively, you can increase the dose as needed if you also want to target other health issues or symptoms (see chapter relating to your specific issue).
- If you experience a THC side effect like intoxication, increased heart rate or anxiety, refer to Chapter Five for how to deal with THC side effects to assess how to continue (and also let your doctor know that you have experienced this side effect).

Look for these beneficial terpenes and minor cannabinoids:

- Alpha-pinene – may help with memory specifically
- Beta-caryophyllene – anti-inflammatory.
- THCV is an appetite suppressant (no munchies!) and may help regulate a healthy metabolism (i.e. anti-obesity and anti-type 2 diabetes,[20] two things that can detrimentally affect brain ageing).

In addition, these tips are worth considering:

- Consider a long-acting slow-release product such as a transdermal patch to avoid THC highs and lows.
- If you are using cannabis as part of your evening wind-down routine, look for a product rich in myrcene, a sedating, calming terpene.

How to use vaporising cannabis flowers for brain wellness

- Start with high-CBD, low-THC flowers, especially if you have never had THC before (i.e. you are 'cannabis naive').
- If you are experienced with THC, you can try a strain with more THC, known as a balanced strain, but be cautious of potential for intoxication or impairment within a few hours of vaporising, as everyone's reaction is different.
- Start with a matchstick-head-sized amount, especially if it is a strain with more THC.

Choosing a strain for vaporising to start with

Choose strains high in CBD and low in THC. A good starting ratio of CBD to THC is between 15:1 and 20:1 such as:
- Avidekel. This is approximately 15–18% CBD, 0.8–1% THC.
- ACDC. This is a very high-CBD, low-THC strain, up to 20% CBD and around 1% or less THC (average CBD to THC ratio is 24:1).

- Cannatonic. This strain can have THC levels up to 6%, which is a bit high, but the way it is grown and the specific subtype makes a difference. If you choose this strain, make sure the THC levels are 3% or below ideally, and CBD content is 10% or higher.
- Any CBD cultivar. Technically, any strain of cannabis can be bred into a high-CBD strain, including strains that were originally higher in THC – they breed out a large amount of the THC. There is no standard term for these high-CBD strains, but they are known by labels such as CBD cultivars or CBD flowers (when it's a dried cannabis product).

Neurological disorders

Understanding what happens and why when things go wrong in the brain in neurodegenerative diseases, especially in Parkinson's and dementia, is not just a professional interest for me, it's also extremely close to home. I watched my dad battle a terrible neurodegenerative brain disease for many years in the time before I knew anything about cannabis and CBD. What was first diagnosed as severe post-concussion syndrome after a major car accident got better at first and his life returned almost to normal. Except that it never quite did. He never felt quite well or the same as before, and my mum noticed it too; small things at first that could be overlooked easily.

Next there was the diagnosis of mild cognitive impairment, which eventually turned into a full-blown aggressive neurodegenerative disease, possibly triggered by a series of injuries over the years, as well as other possible risk factors like his family history of dementia, possible high exposure to agricultural chemicals when he was younger, and maybe even dry-cleaning chemicals. The list of potential risk factors was very long and frustratingly hard to untangle. Dad eventually developed a complex neurodegenerative disorder, including a type of dementia that would at first slowly and then quite quickly rob him of both his body and brain function, as well as features of Parkinsonism, hallucinations and delirium.

It was heartbreaking to see my smart, funny dad, who loved people, his work and life in general, lose his abilities one by one, as his world grew smaller and smaller. He eventually lost the ability to talk and even swallow. I'd suspected there was a problem many years before he received anything diagnosable, even before I was a medical student. However, for years I was told repeatedly by the best specialists that there was nothing wrong, and then, when it was clear there was an issue, that there was nothing that could be done. If I had known then what I know now, I would have had him doing neurofeedback brain training after his severe concussions as part of his recovery, and I also would have had him on a cannabis medicine from day one of his recovery, over 20 years before the onset of his finally diagnosed terminal illness.

If my dad had had access to cannabis as a medicine, as well as all the other brain health tools I have now, who knows, he might still be alive today, or at the very least have had a better quality of life in his final years. When he was first experiencing very early symptoms of cognitive changes, back in 2001, medical cannabis was already a possibility in Canada, but no doctors spoke of it, let alone dared to recommend it. Most never even knew it existed as an option. Back then, even though it was technically legal for someone to use cannabis for a medical reason, it just wasn't an option in reality. Thankfully, we have come a long way in the past 20 years, and there is now a growing evidence base that, far from being a dangerous and toxic drug for the brain, it is actually neuroprotective, especially the lower-THC, higher-CBD varieties. This means that when used in the right way, it can actually protect the adult brain and nervous system from a variety of toxic insults and may even be able to slow down processes associated with the premature deterioration of the brain.

The endocannabinoid system in neurodegenerative brain diseases

The endocannabinoid system has become of keen interest as a treatment target in diseases like Alzheimer's and Parkinson's. This is because these brain diseases involve changes in our cannabinoid receptors.[21] One example of these changes is the loss of CB1 receptors and making too many CB2 receptors.[22] Too many CB2 receptors may be related to a dysfunctional immune system component in these diseases. We also now know, as mentioned earlier, that amyloid plaque build-up in Alzheimer's is likely an immune response, and multiple sclerosis is an immune dysfunction disease of the brain and nervous system too. In both cases, cannabinoids like CBD and THC from the plant that work on our endocannabinoid system seem to help the symptoms of the disease, and may even hold promise for a treatment or cure in the future. CB1 receptors appear to be neuroprotective,[23] so if they start to disappear, that's a sign something is amiss.

Multiple sclerosis

Experts are still debating whether MS is primarily a brain degenerative disease triggered by inflammation or should be thought of as a primary autoimmune disease. It's really just semantics, because MS is actually both. It is an autoimmune disease where the brain and nervous system attacks itself (the nerve sheaths in particular). It can also be thought of as a neurodegenerative disease in that it causes degeneration or breakdown of the fatty nerve sheaths, causing nerve damage. This is a process called demyelination, which means the disease strips from the sensitive nerve fibres the fatty protective sheath that allows nerves to transmit signals to each other for normal brain and nervous system function.

In a form of MS called primary progressive, the degeneration is severe and fast, while other milder forms can be stable for many years before they progress again. Symptoms of MS can vary widely, which often leads to them occurring for years before a diagnosis is received. They can include pain, fatigue, weakness or numbness in various parts of the body, vision problems, dizziness, problems with walking and balance, bowel and bladder problems and muscle spasticity. These can come on without warning, causing extreme pain and disability during attacks.

We now know that MS involves dysregulation of the endocannab-inoid system.[24, 25, 26, 27, 28] Like the other neuropathological brain diseases discussed in this chapter, there is no known pharmaceutical drug cure, and even the best available Western medicine treatments are usually inadequate at controlling symptoms.

According to multiple studies and large data reviews, as well as clinical evidence with many thousands of patients, cannabis has what we classify as strong evidence for helping with something called spasticity, one of the main symptoms of MS. Spasticity is a very disabling symptom that causes muscles and limbs to feel heavy, difficult to move and uncomfortable and in some cases to actually go into painful spasms. In general, it is THC that has the antispasmodic effect (anti-spasticity), but using a good amount of CBD buffers possible THC side effects, including possible effects of high THC on cognition and memory, both of which are already an issue in MS.

Both CBD and THC decrease inflammatory chemicals in the brain microglia (helper cells).[29] That is probably an important effect too, because brain inflammation plays a significant role in the disease process and seems to drive progression (i.e. making the disease worse over time).[30]

Some researchers believe that CBD in very high doses (above the average medical cannabis doses used) may actually be able to at least slow down,[31] or maybe even halt the disease process through its anti-inflammatory action. Sativex, a pharmaceutical cannabis medicine spray made from the plant material that contains an even 1:1 ratio of THC:CBD, is approved for use in MS in the UK and many other EU countries, as well as in Australia, Canada and Israel. This medication is a great option for many people and a huge step that this is now an accepted treatment option which I too have prescribed to some of my patients. However it has been my experience that most of my patients preferred the full spectrum cannabis oils and vaporised flower products, partially due to cost (medical cannabis was far cheaper than the drug, at least in Canada) and also the level of individual tailoring we could accomplish by adjusting CBD to THC ratios and using different strains to vaporise for different types of symptoms, such as the fatigue and depression that many people with MS suffer with. Having as many cannabinoid medicine options for patients as possible is the name of the game and I suspect pharma cannabinoid drugs made from the plant will grow in number and variety as the science of cannabis advances, a trend hopefully all patients will benefit from.

Multiple studies have proven cannabis in various forms to be helpful and effective for many symptoms of MS, including pain and fatigue. In my clinical experience, I have found it useful for these symptoms and also for helping improve quality of life, sleep and anxiety and depression associated with MS, decreasing side effects of medications and reducing the doses of many medications needed. I have treated MS patients whose symptoms improved quite dramatically and whose attacks seemed less frequent after taking medical cannabis consistently over many months.

Using cannabis and CBD in MS

These are general guidelines only, based on what I have found works best for my MS patients:

- Daytime base: high-CBD, low-THC oil, tincture or capsule. I usually start with a high-CBD, low-THC oral or sublingual product as the base of therapy for the daytime, taken 3x/day with meals. You can try using hemp-based CBD oil, but with my patients in Canada, I normally use a medical strain by prescription that contains around 0.5–2% THC, or a 20:1 ratio CBD to THC product, starting at 5–10 mg/dose and slowly increasing the dose for symptom relief. Look for a product labelled as hybrid or sativa-dominant with a variety of terpenes good for inflammation (beta-caryophyllene) and for mood-lifting (D-limonene) as well as alpha-pinene for memory.
- Night-time pain and insomnia and muscle spasms: I normally start with a micro dose (1–2 mg) of a higher-THC, low-CBD or 1:1 oil taken an hour before sleep. The THC helps with the sleep disruption, muscle spasm and pain.

- For immediate relief of spasticity or fatigue during the day: once you are used to THC (after 2–4 weeks of using the night-time THC-containing oil), try vaporising a balanced strain of dried cannabis (see Chapter Five).

Parkinson's disease

As with other neurodegenerative disorders, Parkinson's and similar disorders involve the endocannabinoid system. Cannabinoids are a promising treatment, especially since the best conventional drug therapy options are limited, do not slow disease progression and often do not adequately manage symptoms or improve quality of life to a great degree. The early published research for using cannabis medicines to treat Parkinson's is promising, and the number of positive studies is increasing each month. Multiple studies have now found symptomatic improvement with medical cannabis,[32] and more and more conventional medicine neurologist specialists are considering this option for their patients.[33]

One recent study found that many Parkinson's patients were already trying cannabis as a self-treatment approach,[34] although not always sharing this information with their doctors, and that they found it helpful for a variety of symptoms including tremor, rigidity and other movement and gait problems, depression, anxiety, sleep and pain, with oils seeming to work the best, with least side effects, and vaporising working fastest for tremor relief.

The research is starting to reflect my clinical experience that high CBD medical cannabis is often able to help an immense amount with the non-tremor symptoms of Parkinson's: sleep disturbance, behavioural symptoms ranging from mild to psychosis, and overall quality of life.[35]

I have found a higher success rate than the reported statistics by tweaking the CBD to THC ratio and testing different products under close supervision over a period of months. For example, for self-treatment without guidance from a doctor, some of the most common reported side effects were forgetfulness and dizziness, both things that can be minimised with careful micro-dosing and building the doses very slowly, since the disease makes people's nervous systems extremely sensitive to change.

Anything you add to a person's medication, including something natural like cannabis, must be done with extreme caution and patience, using the 'start low, go slow' approach. I have also found that sticking to high-CBD, low THC products during the day works best, while reserving the higher-THC products for help with sleep disturbance and restlessness, including restless leg syndrome, which is often an issue seen in those diagnosed with Parkinson's and similar disorders.

Too much daytime THC, especially if the dose is too high too soon, can impair balance and co-ordination and change the muscle rigidity too fast, making the muscles overly relaxed and unable to help support walking. Especially in the first few weeks of starting medical cannabis, it is important to watch for low blood pressure, as cannabis slightly lowers blood pressure and people with Parkinson's often already have trouble keeping their blood pressure within the normal range, making them at risk of fainting and falls.

Depression as a result of Parkinson's effects on the brain's mood balance is a very common symptom, and often under-recognised or under-treated. I have found it to respond quite well to cannabis, although finding the best product and strain sometimes takes a few tries. This symptom contributes hugely to the loss of quality of life, because it worsens the social isolation and despair imposed by the disease.

One of the things that led me into integrative medicine, and cannabis medicine within it, was the focus on quality of life. This is especially true in cases where we cannot cure but we can still provide comfort and ease suffering, including helping to alleviate depression. The improvement in mood and depression with cannabis has been one of the most profound changes I have seen with my patients. After adding cannabis, they become less withdrawn and are able to connect again with their loved ones and carers. This connection is often disrupted in Parkinson's because the disease causes loss of facial expression – the 'masked' face, where smiling becomes harder and harder.

Using cannabis and CBD in Parkinson's disease

These are general guidelines only, based on what I have found works best for my Parkinson's patients:

- Daytime base: high-CBD, low-THC oil is best, due to being slower-release (and therefore less likely to cause low blood pressure) and easier to take than capsules (for those with problems swallowing). I usually start with a high-CBD, low-THC oil as the base of therapy for the daytime, taken 2–3x/day with meals. You can try using hemp-based CBD oil, or if available, such as I do in Canada with my patients, try a medical strain by prescription that contains around 0.5–1% THC, or a 20–25:1 ratio CBD to THC product, starting at 5 mg/dose and slowly increasing for symptom relief, checking for side effects such as dizziness, low blood pressure and worsening thinking or confusion. Look for a product with a variety of terpenes good for inflammation (beta-caryophyllene) and for depression (D-limonene) as well as alpha-pinene for memory.
- Night-time pain and insomnia and muscle spasms: I normally start with a micro dose of 1 mg of a higher-THC or 1:1 CBD to THC oil taken an hour before sleep for help with sleep/ wake-cycle disruption, night discomfort and general restlessness and restless legs syndrome.
- For immediate relief of tremor during the day: once used to THC (after 2–4 weeks of using the night-time THC-containing oil), try vaporising a balanced strain of dried cannabis (see Chapter Five), as long as blood pressure is stable (best to avoid if at risk of fainting).

Alzheimer's disease and dementia

The increase in life span we have seen over the last century or so is of course an enormous 'win' for humans, considering that for 99% of human history our lifespan was less than 18 years, according to ger-ontologist Dr Ken Dychtwald. Nonetheless, this extended lifespan has brought with it new health issues only seen in later adulthood. These issues usually affect people in their sixties and older, although genetic and environmental factors may cause brain health issues to emerge earlier. The most well-known and feared of these brain ageing diseases is Alzheimer's. In addition, there are various other related diseases that lead to the final common result of dementia, such as Lewy body dementia (which my dad suffered with as well as Parkinson's) and vascular dementia (which is like the heart disease of the brain and is strongly influenced by lifestyle factors like poor diet and smoking).

Recent estimates for the UK reveal that almost a million people have dementia,[36] or 1 in 14 people aged 65 or over. In the US, the stats for 2019 are for Alzheimer's alone.[37] It may be the single most costly and difficult health issue facing the baby boomer generation, and there is still no cure or clear prevention strategy. More and more research, however, is pointing to (you guessed it!) the endocannabinoid system as well as immune system dysfunction playing a role.

From an integrative medicine approach to dementias in general, and Alzheimer's in particular, it seems that the earlier you start to intervene with natural non-pharmaceutical drugs, the better. These may delay or slow down the progress of the disease or even, possibly, reverse early changes, as Dr Dale Bredesen is showing with his ground-breaking research focusing on changeable lifestyle and metabolic factors like diet, supplementation and stress hormone and inflammation levels.

Cannabis, especially high-CBD varieties, is in the same category as other natural medicines in terms of an integrative medicine preventative strategy for cognitive (thinking and memory) decline and dementia. If you are experiencing mild cognitive changes that are not yet dementia, than refer to the brain wellness section of this chapter for how you might introduce CBD and medical cannabis for brain health and neuroprotection.

If you (or a loved one) are already in the more advanced stages of Alzheimer's or another dementia, cannabis can still offer relief. I have used cannabis medicine, in oil form, to help patients with the behavioural, mood and sleep changes seen in dementia and also to help with chronic pain when patients who already suffer with chronic pain then develop dementia as well. It's a holistic way to help ease multiple symptoms in a patient who may not always be able to tell you what hurts, or explain in detail why they can't sleep or self-regulate. It can also sometimes help boost appetite to support physical strength and fitness as much as possible.

Much like in other neurodegenerative diseases, the research on cannabis in Alzheimer's is early but promising. That being said, there are reports as far back as the Victorian era of its use in the treatment of dementia. The president of the British Medical Association and doctor to the royal household, Sir John Reynolds, wrote a paper in the *Lancet* (one of the world's most respected medical journals both then and now) all the way back in 1890 advocating the medical use of cannabis,[38] telling of his thirty years of prescribing it for conditions ranging from migraines and nerve pain to – you guessed it – 'senile dementia', aka Alzheimer's.

More recently, both lab studies and human studies are showing evidence that cannabis can help with dementia. A number of studies have now shown that multiple cannabinoids and other cannabis plant chemicals such as cannflavin A have the ability to get rid of the beta-amyloid plaques that build up in the brain in Alzheimer's,[39, 40] something that no pharmaceutical drug has been able to accomplish so far. Another study points to the anti-Alzheimer's effects of CBD.[41] It's still early days in terms of translating this into working in humans and finding the right combination of cannabinoids and doses, but it is very exciting, and in time will possibly lead to more effective treatments at the very least.

On a more practical level, multiple studies have now shown that cannabis can be used to effectively treat the behavioural symptoms of dementia as well as low appetite,[42] while another study using a medical cannabis oil of approximately 2:1 CBD to THC ratio found that not only did behavioural symptoms improve with the oil, but also patients' body rigidity (Parkinsonism).[43] There was less of a need for medications, including opioids, which often worsen memory, mood and balance, and may cause severe bowel issues like constipation. In contrast, cannabis was very well tolerated in these patients. More and more doctors are considering adding it to their toolbox for patients in nursing home care who often have dementia as well as other painful chronic conditions.[44]

Even more cautiously positive reports from the research have declared that although we still lack large randomised controlled studies, the risk and adverse effects are low for use in dementia, especially with few other effective options.[45] In reality, since cannabis is a complex botanical medicine, it may be that we are never going to see randomised placebo-controlled trials in exactly the same way that we test a pharma drug, or that the cannabinoid derived drugs take another decade for RCT studies to be done and published. To wait another five or ten years for them is a huge disservice to people who could benefit now from this option for so many symptoms in conditions where drugs fall short and suffering is high.

Using cannabis and CBD in Alzheimer's disease and dementia

These are general guidelines only, based on what I have found works best for my patients incorporating cannabis for management of dementia symptoms. I recommend working with a doctor who specialises in the use of medical cannabis.

- Daytime base: high-CBD, low-THC oil or capsules are best, due to being slower-release than inhaled products. I usually start with a high-CBD, low-THC oil as the base of therapy for the daytime, taken 2–3x/day with meals. You can try using hemp-based CBD oil, or if available, such as I do in Canada with my patients, try a medical strain by prescription that contains around 0.5–1% THC, or a 20–25:1 ratio CBD to THC product, starting at 5–10 mg/dose and slowly increasing the dose for symptom relief, checking for side effects such as dizziness, low blood pressure and worsening thinking or confusion. Look for a product with a variety of terpenes good for inflammation (beta-caryophyllene) and depression (D-limonene) as well as alpha-pinene for memory.

- Night-time pain and insomnia and muscle spasms: I normally start with a micro dose of 1–2 mg of a higher-THC or 1:1 CBD to THC oil or capsule taken an hour before sleep for help with sleep/wake-cycle disruption, what is known as 'sundowning' behaviour, when people become agitated just before sunset, and any other co-occurring pain or night-time discomforts. I have found that a small amount of THC before bed allows patients to discontinue other sleeping pills such as antipsychotic drugs, often used in dementia when other drugs fail. These sleeping pills and antipsychotics have a high side-effect profile and often make the memory, confusion and dementia symptoms worse, so anything that can minimise their use is helpful.

Post-concussion syndrome

This is quite a common syndrome that can result from a seemingly mild knock to the head, even when a brain CT and MRI scan are normal. This is often the case when someone doesn't fully pass out or lose consciousness at the time of the injury, or if multiple small concussions happen over time without anything major showing up on a scan. The symptoms can be very vague and last for months and even years after the head injury. They range from headaches to chronic fatigue and brain fog, agitation and problems with mood stability in a previously well-adjusted person. Patients come to see me with this issue, as do clients at our brain-based wellness centre in Bali, saying that they just can't put their finger on it but they never quite felt the same since their injury, or that they started to improve but don't have the mental bandwidth or stamina they once had. It is incredibly frustrating because no MRI scans or blood tests show up as abnormal and doctors usually tell them they will just have to live with it.

If that sounds familiar, adding in cannabis in the way described in the brain wellness section here can be helpful, along with other brain-support supplements and lifestyle changes, such as taking up a simple meditation practice daily. You can try adding a CBD oil or product (and if chronic fatigue, headaches, anxiety, mood balance or other specific symptoms are a problem, refer to the chapter dealing with that issue). Alongside CBD we have also found that neurofeed-back brain training can help the brain return to a state of equilibrium when other methods have failed.

CHAPTER EIGHT

OVERCOMING STRESS, BURNOUT AND FATIGUE

Stress is a part of life, but the type of chronic unremitting low-level stress we experience in modern life can wreak havoc on our nervous system, our ability to make energy and generally our entire being. Our brains and bodies were designed and evolved to cope with acute danger and short-lived stresses, such as running away from a tiger and then chilling out after the danger had passed. In fact, animals in the wild don't suffer from chronic stress diseases the way us humans do because they process threats differently in the brain. They get over a stressful event quickly after the danger has passed without getting stuck in a stress spiral.[1] Nowadays, the constant daily mental threats we experience are harder for the nervous system to cope with and can throw our stress system and our endocannabinoid system into havoc, causing both brain and body changes that can leave us feeling drained, tired, irritable and brain-foggy.

CBD and cannabis can be very useful tools to help bring us back into balance. Because the endocannabinoid system is intricately involved in coping with chronic stress, when it loses balance, plant cannabinoids can be a great help. But before we get into how to use cannabis and CBD for stress, burnout and chronic fatigue, it's important to understand what burnout actually is and how it affects us.

Burnout syndrome and toxic stress

The World Health Organization now recognises burnout syndrome as a diagnosable medical illness. It might sound like something only overpaid business executives experience, but this level of extreme stress is no joke and the number of people suffering from burnout is rising. For the past half a decade much of my work has been devoted to helping people (and organisations) recover from burnout. I had to deal with a mild form of it myself – twice, actually, since being a triple type A personality, I didn't learn the first time! This chapter could be a whole book in itself, but I will focus mainly on cannabis and CBD and a few other pearls from the programme I use with people suffering from burnout, chronic fatigue and toxic stress. As with other health issues, cannabis and CBD are not an instant cure-all for burnout and chronic fatigue (or a cure for anything for that matter!) but part of a considered holistic approach. However, I consider their use one of my most valuable tools to help people regain balance in these conditions and reduce symptoms to allow recovery to start, especially when many other attempts have failed.

So what exactly is burnout syndrome?

Burnout syndrome is defined by researchers as a state of mental and/or physical exhaustion caused by excessive and prolonged stress. It can also be defined as a constellation of symptoms resulting from the long-term effects of chronic unchecked bad stress on the brain and body. These can range from constant fatigue despite getting 8 hours of sleep, anxiety and low mood to symptoms like feeling less motivated, more cynical and less fulfilled in your work life. A researcher called Christina Maslach started to realise this was a growing issue around 25 years ago and created a questionnaire to measure burnout. Now there is an entire medical research journal (a doctor and researcher magazine if you will!) dedicated to burnout syndrome. We are constantly connected to our devices and have less time for brain and body rest as well as restorative sleep. When this is combined with our brains being overstimulated by screen time and the work culture pressure to be more productive at all costs, it creates the perfect storm of conditions for a burnout epidemic.

Anyone can get burnout. I've treated clients from stay-at-home mums to corporate executives and doctors. After you have had it once, you are more likely to have another burnout, so it's really important to break the cycle once and for all. This is where cannabis and CBD may be able to help.

What burnout looks like: the 3 stages

Stage 1 is known as the stress arousal phase, where the adrenal glands may be pumping out more and more stress hormone and the whole nervous system goes into high-alert mode, leading to symptoms such as irritability, insomnia, forgetfulness, heart palpitations, inability to concentrate and distractibility. Patients may have periods of more energy than normal. They may become super-sensitive to caffeine, and find that it gives them palpitations or makes them wired, though this is then followed by a crash.

Stage 2 is known as the energy conservation phase, where the nervous system and cells are losing steam and measures are taken to conserve both brain and body energy. The brain goes into withdraw and protect mode, leading to issues like procrastination, three-day weekends needed to recover for the next work week, decreased sexual desire, persistent tiredness in the mornings, social withdrawal from friends and/or family, increased need for caffeine just to feel normal, cynical or resentful feelings at work or feeling less satisfaction from your work (if the burnout is work-related), a mix of feeling anxious and then depressed (roller coaster of moods).

Stage 3 is known as the exhaustion phase, where the body's stress coping systems and adrenal glands cannot keep up and cortisol can become too low on functional medicine tests, as opposed to too high as it is in stage 1. This can cause an increasing global unshakeable fatigue and brain depression to set in, as well as problems in other body systems like the gut and symptoms such as chronic sadness or depression, chronic stomach or bowel problems, including IBS type symptoms, waking up feeling exhausted even after 8 hours or more of sleep, chronic persistent daily mental and/or physical fatigue, chronic daily headaches, receiving a diagnosis of chronic fatigue syndrome (CFS) or ME.

CFS/ME is often associated with burnout but can also be triggered by a viral fever in someone who was completely well. It is a complex nervous system, immune system and mitochondria (cell energy) disorder, but cannabis and CBD as well as the other supplements and suggestions in this chapter are still good tools to start with. Leaky gut can also be a factor in CFS/ME, and toxic-stress-induced burnout syndrome in some cases too. So healing the gut is also important for many people and something that should be assessed by a health practitioner familiar with gut health and integrative or functional medicine (also see Chapter Fifteen).

Good stress vs bad stress

Good stress is experienced when stress is limited to a short amount of time and the experience leaves us with a sense of accomplishment, exhilaration or mastery, like the physical stress of running a race, or speaking in public for the first time and getting a positive response from the audience.

Bad stress, on the other hand, is prolonged, emotionally draining and/or physically exhausting and eventually even dangerous to our nervous system and immune system. This kind of unremitting stress starts to wreak havoc on our hormone balance and endocannabinoid system balance. It can trigger a host of problems, such as:

- chronic fatigue
- insomnia
- brain fog

- frequent infections and taking longer than average to recover
- poor memory and trouble retaining information
- anxiety symptoms for no reason, or new onset of depression
- autoimmune issues

Some stress actually improves performance ...

Way back in 1908, two smarty-pants psychologists figured out the relationship between stress levels and our performance, and that some degree of stress actually improves how we function both mentally and physically – it's about getting the right level of good stress and making sure it doesn't turn into the bad kind. This rule was named after them as the Yerkes–Dodson law.

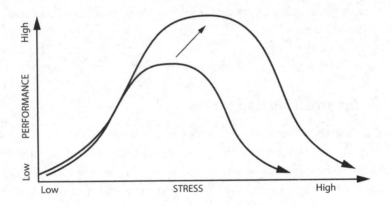

This model shows that there is a level of stress at which a person performs best both mentally and physically. This sweet spot where stress is a good thing is what I like to call the thrive zone. But if you pile up more and more constant chronic stress, the stress burden becomes too high for our balancing systems in the brain and body to cope, and good stress starts to turn into bad stress, resulting in symptoms of burnout.

Using tools including CBD and cannabis medicine as part of a holistic anti-burnout programme can actually change how much stress your brain can handle while still remaining in your thrive zone. Recent research is now supporting the idea that CBD may be able to reduce the total stress burden (called the allostatic load),[2] which can become so high it leads to dysfunction, either burnout or, in the extreme, conditions like PTSD, where the nervous system loses the ability to calm itself down.

Tests on mice seem to demonstrate that CBD's ability to reduce stress is due to its effect on neurogenesis in the brain's hippocampus[3] – i.e. building new neurons in this area[4] involved in memory and stress regulation. Our endocannabinoid system (ECS) is also involved with encoding and influencing our memories associated with stress[5] and changing how we remember stressful experiences. So balancing it using tools like CBD means being able to function at our peak mentally, physically and emotionally under more stress without getting burnout or chronic fatigue by optimising our stress response and expanding our thrive zone.

The Western medicine approach to burnout: there's nothing wrong with you

Scientists have been aware of this stress performance curve for more than a hundred years. Dozens more studies exist proving the detrimental effect of chronic stress on both physical and mental health, yet most medical doctors still haven't got the memo about burnout syndrome and how to treat it. They will often give advice such as 'just take a holiday', or 'stress is normal, everyone has it so we just have to get on with it'. Blood tests come back as normal and the patient is then told that 'nothing is wrong with you' or there is no such thing as burnout syndrome, adrenal fatigue or chronic fatigue – it's all psychological. That's because what we are taught in medical school about these issues, just like what we are taught about cannabis medicine and the endocannabinoid system, is simply out of date. This is a very frustrating journey for people with burnout and is the story of literally every single patient who finds their way to me. I'm often the first medical person they have seen who 'gets it' and doesn't think they are crazy or exaggerating. It's a huge emotional relief to have your symptoms recognised, especially because there is something you can do about it – burnout is not a life sentence!

Annette's story

Many patients who came to see me in my practice were suffering from severe, debilitating burnout and/or chronic fatigue. For them, adding cannabis medicine was the catalyst they needed to get their lives back. Annette was one of these people. She was referred to see me for a list of problems she herself described as 'a mile long'. She had seen every specialist under the sun and had been diagnosed with chronic fatigue syndrome, depression, anxiety, insomnia, IBS and some chronic pain conditions as well. She was on a mountain of drugs for these ailments, and then more drugs for the side effects of the original ones. Despite maximum medical therapy, she wasn't any better. She had also tried therapy after being told by one doctor, 'It's all in your head.'

But when I interviewed Annette for the first time, it was clear that, far from being negative about the world or wanting to give up on life, she was frustrated by not having the energy to do what she wanted. I felt that chronic fatigue and burnout were a more accurate diagnosis than just depression, although she certainly had symptoms consistent with depression as part of her burnout. When I told her this, she was very hopeful and excited because she didn't feel depressed, although she found having no energy was depressing – a normal reaction, we all can agree!

We started a high-CBD, low-THC oil daily and also added a micro dose of a THC oil for her sleep at night. After six weeks, she was much better and sleeping more deeply but still 'felt like a truck had hit her' when she woke up and was taking a few hours to get going (one of the reasons she had to quit her job and go on disability, since this meant she often had to call in sick or be very late). We added a very small dose of 1–2 vaporised inhalations of a sativa-dominant balanced product first thing in the morning, which did not make her feel high or impaired but helped activate her nervous system normally for the first time in over five years. To Annette, it felt like a miracle, especially because she had tried so many drugs and pills that had failed her.

Burnout can sneak up on you

Burnout is one of those issues that can happen in different ways: slowly over years of chronic stress you barely notice, or like a ton of bricks that hits you one day so that you suddenly collapse from exhaustion seemingly out of nowhere, often after a big life stressor. When chronic fatigue is the main issue, it may start with a virus. In my own case, I contracted dengue fever for the second time when in Bali (the first time was in Thailand six years previous to that), and the weeks after the virus left me with debilitating brain fog and fatigue. Luckily I was able to treat these symptoms successfully using all the tools in this chapter, and was back to 100% in less than three months. If I had not been able to dedicate myself completely to my recovery, I believe I could have ended up in bed for three years, like some of my clients who were suffering from post-virus chronic fatigue syndrome before they got to me. Other people with chronic fatigue illness improve once the leaky gut issue is dealt with, something integrative medicine doctors have noted for years, but only recently has there been published preliminary evidence for this.[6]

But no matter what triggers a burnout or chronic fatigue illness, nothing is scarier than going almost overnight from being an energetic, high-functioning human to bed-bound and unable to remember what you read an hour before. The upside of experiencing this myself is that I have gained a deep understanding of what my clients and patients go through and how to help them get their life back, beat burnout and regain their energy levels and stress resilience.

What actually happens in burnout: the brain loses its off switch

I always start by explaining to someone with burnout that it's as if a circuit-breaker in the brain that controls things like energy levels and brain function gets flipped the wrong way and you can't seem to turn it back on. Or another way of putting it: the brain gets stuck in constant hyper-vigilance, or fight-or-flight mode, and loses its off switch. When I question new patients with burnout about how they are winding down, relaxing, letting go, and ask, 'So how's your off switch?' they often respond completely seriously, 'What off switch?'

When your sympathetic fight-or-flight mode is on all the time, it tells the hypothalamus part of your brain to instruct your adrenal glands to pump out more stress hormone chemicals, such as cortisol. Those same stress hormones loop back around and hang out in the brain, activating the amygdala (the part of your brain that increases the intensity of sadness, fear and anger emotions) and blocking the brain from laying down new learning and memories in the hippocampus. This also unbalances your endocannabinoid system, which we are now discovering helps control the stress response via the HPA axis (see below)[7] and cortisol through brain receptors in the hypothalamus area of the brain. The chronic unchecked fight-or-flight mode actually physically changes the brain areas that control and rein in the stress response, such as the hippocampus, the amygdala and the VMPFC (ventral medial prefrontal cortex). These changes can be so significant that they can actually be seen on an MRI scan.

So needless to say, helping to restore the balance in the brain by modulating the ECS (and therefore our stress response) using CBD[8] and cannabinoids from the cannabis plant is incredibly promising. Using CBD to help do this is also very safe, since it seems that this modulation effect can work without needing THC onboard. Groundbreaking research in mice has concluded that CBD on its own has the ability to control the stress response via the HPA axis by acting on a type of serotonin receptor called 5-HTR1A.

Another factor in burnout and across the chronic fatigue spectrum (including CFS/ME) is thought to be related to our cell energy powerhouses, known as mitochondria, becoming dysfunctional and not producing cell energy normally. Cannabinoids are also regulators of these mitochondria energy factories in every one of our cells, as well as regulating a brain protein called BDNF (brain-derived neurotrophic factor),[9] in charge of making new brain cells and enhancing brain function as well as protecting the brain from toxins and injury. This may be why so many people who try CBD wellness products even at low doses report a huge shift in their energy levels and mental clarity – these are also basically brain anti-ageing plant chemicals too!

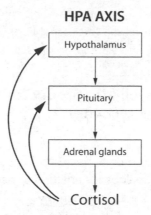

HPA AXIS

HPA stands for hypothalamic–pituitary–adrenal, and this axis is the main brain-controlled pathway for releasing stress hormones from the adrenal glands, which sit on top of the kidneys. The endocannabinoid system is involved with regulation of the HPA axis at a brain level.

CBD to the rescue: anti-burnout adaptogen

As we touched on in Chapter One, cannabis can be considered a power plant, with potent effects on our brain and body even at relatively small doses. But unlike the other power plants mentioned, cannabis, and especially high-CBD, low-THC products, can be used to help restore homeostasis and help balance our stress response system. That is because one of our endocannabinoid system's jobs is to balance stress, and CBD and other chemicals in the cannabis plant seem to work with our ECS to help it do this. In botanical medicine, plant medicines that work in our bodies to help them adapt better to chronic stress are known as adaptogens. They can help us regulate our cortisol, or stress hormone, levels. In order to qualify as adaptogens, they must also be safe (low toxicity), non-intoxicating and non-addictive, all boxes that CBD ticks.

In addition to high-CBD cannabis products and hemp-based CBD wellness products, I also routinely recommend other adaptogens to help the body restore balance and manage stress. These include an Indian herb called ashwagandha, different forms and combinations of medicinal mushrooms (chaga, reishi, cordyceps, lion's mane) and Chinese herbs such as schisandra and eleutherococcus, to name just a few.

How to use CBD wellness products (hemp CBD) for burnout and stress recovery

- Try a full-spectrum (or broad-spectrum) CBD oil.
- If fatigue is a big issue, look for uplifting terpenes:
    - alpha-pinene – good for memory
    - D-limonene – smells like lemons and has both anti-anxiety and antidepressant effects so is thought of as a mood-balancing terpene.

Starting dose and titrating up

Try 10 mg of CBD first thing in the morning, at midday/early afternoon (12–2 p.m.) and at dinner time for a total of 30 mg/day. Stay at this dose for 1–2 weeks and track your symptoms to test how you feel:

- Is the stress level improving?
- Is the fatigue improving?
- How about other symptoms, like irritability, brain fog, feeling overwhelmed?
- How about mood?
- Is it still bad at a certain time of day?
- Are you still having trouble getting to sleep or staying asleep?

Score your energy level each day in the morning, afternoon and evening (after dinner) on a scale from 0 to 10, where 0 = no anxiety, 10 = unbearable/worst anxiety imaginable, and write down the results in your symptom tracker.

You can slowly increase the dose each week, keeping in mind that it may take weeks/months to see a full effect. If you reach 60 mg total per day of CBD, stay at this level for another 4–6 weeks before increasing again (since the effects of CBD can take weeks in some people, this will avoid increasing the dose unnecessarily).

Remember: there is no specific perfect dose that works for everyone exactly the same way, because each person's endocannabinoid system and their balance is unique. So self-titration, starting low and slow with your dosing, is the name of the game as to how much CBD to take.

INDICA VS SATIVA

Most strains of hemp CBD oils are hybrids, but if you find the hemp CBD oil you choose is making you feel more fatigued or tired, it may be rich in myrcene, which can be too sedating for daytime use if you have chronic fatigue. Check the label, and if this is the case, change to a different brand and look for one with a terpene profile that is low in myrcene for daytime.

How to use medical cannabis products for burnout, stress and chronic fatigue

Only try this under the supervision of a doctor and, of course, if medical cannabis (containing THC) is legal where you live.

- Start with a high-CBD cannabis oil as your base. This is the best starting product for burnout and chronic fatigue, taken by mouth.
- When it comes to burnout and fatigue and THC, less is more!
- Average starting daytime dose: 5 mg x3/day for a total of 15 mg. The THC dose will depend on the product, but start with 1 mg of daytime THC max (i.e. an oil that has a THC to CBD ratio of 1:20 will give you 1 mg of THC for every 20 mg of CBD).

- Keep increasing the dose until you feel the symptoms improving.
- Because most people with burnout and chronic fatigue have 'tired but wired' systems, especially in stage 1 and stage 2, sleep is often disrupted even though they are overtired, with non-restorative light sleep and a lack of deep sleep. For these sleep issues, try an additional 2 mg dose of THC an hour before bedtime, using a THC oil labelled as 'indica' and rich in myrcene and CBN (see Chapter Eleven).

How to use vaporising cannabis flowers for burnout syndrome

- Vaporised cannabis can be used as an add-on to oils, either cannabis oils or hemp CBD oils.

Just like with oils, start with high-CBD, low-THC flower. Strains of cannabis with a high CBD to THC around 20:1 include:

- Avidekel. This is approximately 15–18% CBD, 0.8–1% THC.
- ACDC. This is a very high-CBD, low-THC strain, up to 20% CBD and around 1% or less THC (average CBD to THC ratio is 24:1).
- Any CBD cultivar. Technically, any strain of cannabis can be bred into a high-CBD strain, including strains that were originally higher in THC – they breed out a large amount of the THC. There is no standard term for these high-CBD strains, but they are known by labels such as CBD cultivars or CBD flowers (when it's a dried cannabis product).
- If this has no effect, you can try a strain with slightly more THC, such as a 1:5 CBD to THC, or a balanced strain with equal amounts of CBD and THC, i.e. 1:1.
- Start with a matchstick-head-sized amount, especially if it is a strain with more THC.
- Some people find this to be a good substitute for alcohol to help wind down in the evening before doing a meditation or relaxation practice, since I recommend cutting out alcohol and

caffeine completely for three months if you are suffering with burnout or chronic fatigue.

- If anxiety is a major feature of your burnout syndrome, I have also used vaporised high-CBD cannabis to replace prescription anxiety pills and help successfully wean patients off drugs such as benzodiazepines (this should be done under medical supervision by a doctor).

- Cannabis flower can also be used before bedtime to help you get to sleep more easily and wind down a busy mind. Try a strain high in myrcene (see Chapter Eleven) if you only have trouble getting to sleep but have no problems with light sleep, sleep fragmentation or waking up prematurely in the early morning hours (in which cases an oil is best, since it lasts longer).

- One way in which I have found vaporised cannabis extremely useful is in patients with crushing morning fatigue. This has not yet been reported in published literature but it is something I have seen work time and time again, especially since I get a lot of patients referred to me with chronic fatigue. This fatigue can come from a variety of sources, including MS, fibromyalgia and chronic pain, and not much else has helped them – certainly not drugs, although they have tried them all! This morning fatigue robs them of their entire day because it is a struggle to do the simple things needed to get out the door, let alone think of anything more rigorous, like housework, cooking, exercising, socialising or going to work. I tend to look for what is often labelled as a sativa-dominant balanced strain (a THC to CBD ratio of 1:5 to start with), rich in limonene and alpha-pinene, and get them to take 1–2 inhalations first thing, while they are still in bed. This technique is often the energy hack they need to start being able to live some sort of life again. And it also seems that once the brain is more activated, everything starts to get a bit easier and shift in a positive direction.

CHAPTER NINE

ADDRESSING ANXIETY AND PTSD

Anxiety is something most people have experienced at some point in their life. For many, it's a daily companion. Whether it shows up in the form of constriction in your throat, chest tightness, a sensation of not feeling at ease or comfortable in your skin, a general fear kind of feeling or even a dodgy stomach, anxiety is one annoying MF.

So where does it actually come from and why does it seem to be reaching epidemic levels in modern life? Part of it is cultural: we live in a hyper-stimulated, hyper-connected world – endlessly attached to our phones, computers, TVs and social media – yet we are often disconnected from each other in 'real' life.

Our current normal pace of life would have sent our grandparents mad, with many of us cramming more things into one day than they would have done in a week. We are encroaching on our relaxation time for one more hour of productivity, and we do it daily without pause. This has an effect on our nervous system and, you guessed it, on our good old endocannabinoid system, whose job it is to help us relax and protect us from stress and anxiety.

The good news is that no matter where you are right now with anxiety, you can get it under control. And the better news is that CBD and cannabis can help.

Anxiety: the scope of the problem

In the UK alone, recent statistics showed that one in six adults had experienced some form of 'neurotic health problem' (aka anxiety) in the last seven days. Three million people in the UK meet the clinical criteria for an anxiety disorder,[1] which is the most severe level of anxiety. The sheer number of people experiencing symptoms makes anxiety one of the most common issues affecting our well-being, at every stage of life.

Symptoms of anxiety can show up anywhere in the body, in many different ways. Some people may experience it as a sense of being overwhelmed, where little things that should be easy become almost impossible to manage. For others, it can be physical, in the form of a lump in the throat, a racing heart, chest tightness, sweating or a feeling of tunnel vision that can come on randomly without warning. For yet others, it is more cerebral, showing up as a constant mental chatter that is hard or near impossible to block out.

Despite there being more and more anti-anxiety drugs on the market, the problem isn't getting any better. The pill approach to anxiety may be a temporary fix in the short term, but it comes with significant, even scary, side effects and the long-term results are disappointing. These drugs unfortunately do little to help the nervous system to regain balance, so you can sometimes need more and more of them to keep functioning, with a nervous system that is still constantly on edge.

Anxiety is often suffered in secret, especially in the wellness community, where people feel they should have it all figured out before they teach others. I actually have hundreds of clients who are wellness practitioners, yoga and meditation teachers and coaches. They still suffer with anxiety and have what I call 'yogic guilt' because they haven't fully cracked their own anxiety, despite teaching techniques to overcome it for a living. But the reality is that beating anxiety is a journey with good days and not-so-good-days and no one is perfectly balanced all of the time. Adding in CBD to their toolkit has helped many practitioners crack that tricky 'in the moment' anxiety that can come on suddenly and needs a quick fix (especially in quick acting vaporised form). All the while, their routine mind-body practices, such as meditation, keep chipping away at the more chronic nervous system wind-up. Some of them have even added it to their practice, and CBD yoga classes are now popping up all over the place for the same reason – it's the perfect companion to yoga and meditation.

When used properly, cannabis and CBD can be an effective way to support a return to a calm, balanced nervous system and, despite the recent concerns about safety from certain regulatory bodies, I still believe it is as safe or safer than many other drugs and supplements for anxiety, especially at the doses most commonly used.

On its own, or better yet combined with some simple relaxation techniques and lifestyle hacks, properly administered CBD and high-CBD, very low-THC medical cannabis can relieve even very intense anxiety. With its help you can reclaim your life from what can be a crippling problem affecting everything from your relationships, work and social life to bodily functions like bowel habits and IBS symptoms. In this way, CBD and medical cannabis can be like a herbal meditation assistant that can help the brain get into a calmer state long enough to start training it with mind-body techniques to reap long-term anxiety-busting benefits.

The integrative medicine view of anxiety

From an integrative medicine point of view, anxiety (and its close cousins depression and burnout) is viewed as a problem of central nervous system regulation. It is an imbalance of the homeostasis needed to maintain a calm nervous system, and an inability to return to baseline after a stressful event jacks up our fight-or-flight system. Essentially, it is a winding-down problem.

The causes are multifactorial, which is a fancy word for saying it's complicated. There is no one cause for anxiety, but the multiple causes include many factors from our high-speed culture, individual personality tendencies, genes, food and the environment.

This process of perpetual wind-up goes on over months and years, gradually changing our brain chemicals, including depleting GABA, which is the calming neurotransmitter chemical. GABA depletion, along with changes related to our other brain chemicals and our endocannabinoid system, leaves us almost perpetually frazzled, and over time our brain pathway changes and we become hard-wired for anxiety. If the process goes unchecked for years at a time, the nervous system ends up in a constant state of hyperarousal. In other words, anxiety becomes our brain's new normal.

How cannabis works on anxiety in our brain

So how does this relate to cannabis and CBD? Well, our endocannabinoid system helps regulate all the brain chemical (neurotransmitter) systems, including GABA. It plays a huge role in rebalancing the wound-up hyper-vigilant nervous system.

Cannabinoids in the brain also decrease our fight-or-flight response,[2] reduce both physical and perceived mental stress and help restore deep sleep. So it all comes back to certain types of cannabis and CBD helping our endocannabinoid system to get back into balance and calm down the nervous system. We need to break what I call the anxiety spirals in the brain, which may involve GABA levels going down, the brain getting stuck on 'go' all the time and the limbic system (our fear and emotional memory brain area) becoming hypersensitive. The brain can start to see everything as a threat (start to feel on edge), deep sleep goes down the toilet and the nervous system wind-up becomes more and more difficult to stop.

Cannabis medicines and wellness products, especially ones high in CBD, can be the catalyst to start reversing these changes. Their immediate effects get you a quick win, and that helps you feel calm enough to be able to convince your brain to start doing (and keep doing!) other really helpful things like meditation and relaxation techniques to break the anxiety cycle for good.

Cannabis and CBD for anxiety 'fails' using recreational dispensaries and shops

With legal recreational cannabis now available to consumers in shops in Canada, some US states, Amsterdam and all of Uruguay, there is a growing issue of people attempting to self-medicate their anxiety. In many cases, they do not have the information or the expertise to successfully match up their symptoms with the right cannabis product from a non-medical dispensary.

I have had many frustrated phone calls from friends, and also heard stories from patients, who have been sold a totally inappropriate cannabis product for their medical or wellness situation, resulting in confusion, accidental THC overuse or just feeling weird.

One friend was told by the well-meaning teenage shop assistant to just dump a bottle of THC tincture into a water bottle and 'drink it as you like'. Unfortunately, my friend had never taken any THC before and had actually asked for a CBD oil for anxiety. The advice led to a full-blown panic attack and a trip to the hospital because she thought she was having a heart attack!

If you have access to lots of cannabis products for anxiety but zero clue where to start, this chapter can hopefully help guide you to find the right product and avoid any cannabis fails.

Alex's story: even meditating makes me anxious

Alex was referred to me for help. She had tried nearly everything to manage her anxiety, which took many forms: general anxiety that was a constant fixture, with additional ramped-up anxiety when she was in a busy public space that sometimes spiralled into full-blown panic attacks. This had led to her leaving the house less and less, becoming more isolated. Ironically, seeking help for her anxiety at the doctor's led to more anxiety attacks when she had to force herself to go to an appointment and sit in the hectic waiting room. It had reached the point where she had missed so many appointments that her doctor threatened to fire her as a patient.

Alex had to rely on benzodiazepines daily, which can cause dependency, only work for a few hours at a time and have lots of side effects, including rebound anxiety and nasty withdrawals. She was also taking an SSRI (a medication from the same family as Prozac used for both anxiety and depression) for the daytime, and on top of that sleeping pills to help her get to sleep and stay asleep. She had struggled with anxiety for as long as she could remember.

Alex had tried meditation, which exacerbated her anxiety so badly she could no longer practise it. This made her especially guilty and discouraged since she was a yoga teacher. She had also done a few courses of cognitive behavioural therapy (CBT), which helped somewhat, but because her nervous system was so on edge most of the time, it was hard to break the anxiety loops in the moment and use her CBT techniques.

She had heard that CBD and medical cannabis might help but was scared to try it on her own due to a bad experience with cannabis as a teenager, when a single joint led to a severe panic attack and she had to go the hospital because she felt like she was dying. It was pretty scary and she was afraid it would happen again if she tried any form of cannabis.

One of her goals, along with getting better control of her anxiety attacks so she could go out socially, was to get off the benzodiazepine pills. She felt she was hooked on them, and she was right, as that is exactly what happens with long-term use of these pills. Her doctor had not told her that was a risk when she started them. Apart from the issue of habituation, relying on the tablets for the rest of her life was not in alignment with her desire for a more natural approach to tackling her anxiety. Then there were the side effects, like withdrawal and inability to think and function if she missed a dose. In addition to the anxiety tablets, she also wanted to get off the sleeping pills. They made her feel funny in the morning, and though they knocked her out most nights, she never felt fully rested. These types of pills interfere with slow-wave sleep,[3] stage 1 and REM sleep,[4] and the scary thing is that many of my new patients, although they have been prescribed these drugs for daily use for years, have never been told this by their doctors. They are usually shocked, angry and confused when they learn about these side effects,[5] and most say they would have never started taking them in the first place if they had known. These patients do, however, still need real help for their sleep, and this is where I believe the right cannabis product provides a low-risk alternative.

The first time I saw Alex, over video telemedicine, she was sitting in her living room with her cat, Max. She confessed right away that even waiting for this appointment had filled her with such anxiety she had almost cancelled it and the only reason she kept it was because she could see me from home and avoid a panic-inducing doctor's office trip.

We started chatting about her cat. I love meeting my patients' pets when I see them over video conference from their homes. It's become a regular part of these types of visits to open by chatting about their animals, who often sit in their laps during the appointment. In addition to being enjoyable, I find it allows me to rapidly develop stronger relationships and rapport with my patients, which contributes to better outcomes.

I dug into a thorough history of Alex's anxiety, her life in general and her health history. After assessing her and hearing her story, we decided that there was no reason not to try cannabis. I assured her that we would use high-CBD, very low-THC forms to avoid having another bad reaction like she had when she was a teen, and that we would monitor things together to find the best strains. I explained that her panic attack was due to her smoking a very high-THC, low-CBD form of cannabis common on the recreational black market, since high doses of THC can actually cause anxiety. On the other hand, micro doses of THC combined with a lot of CBD can be very effective as an anxiety treatment.

I also explained to her that her experience of worsening anxiety with meditation was a known phenomenon in integrative medicine, but that with some coaching, introducing short, simple meditations after taking a dose of her high-CBD oil, I was confident she could overcome this issue and start to enjoy meditation again. This made her very excited and hopeful for the first time in years.

We started Alex on a low-THC, high-CBD oil (25:1 ratio) and a very small dose (2 mg) of THC indica oil for sleep. After six months, she had stopped her benzos, was on the lowest possible dose of the SSRI and had stopped taking sleeping pills. She had been able to get up to a 15-minute meditation practice each day and was actually enjoying it now and starting to find that it calmed her thoughts. She was looking at meditation teacher training courses to enrol in. She was able to leave the house and go out for dinner with her friends, and had even started dating.

Dan's story: the cannabis mystery effect

Dan was referred to me by his GP for help with anxiety but for a slightly different reason. He had been self-medicating his anxiety disorder with recreational cannabis for years, after coming off anxiety medications because of side effects and because he preferred to go natural.

He had been using a combination of black market and home-grown cannabis from friends. This led to a guessing game as to the strain and THC and CBD content. Sometimes he was given the supposed strain name, but this wasn't able to be confirmed by a lab test since it wasn't a regulated medical cannabis product. He had no idea of the amounts of THC and CBD, or whether it contained chemical contaminants and other nasties.

These were all reasons that led him to see me. He wanted to know first of all what he was taking, to make sure it was safe and uncontaminated. Second, he wanted to try to reproduce the same effect every time. He had smoked cannabis for years, and recently changed to vaporising after hearing it was safer than smoking. However, even with vaporising the non-medical cannabis, the results were still hit and miss for his anxiety symptoms. Even when cannabis did work well for Dan's immediate anxiety, sometimes an hour or two later he felt worse than before. So it was a bit like cannabis roulette, gambling as to whether the strain he managed to get hold of would work for his anxiety, how much he would need and what side effects he would experience.

He was also intrigued by the idea of getting legally prescribed medical cannabis using specific strains and dosages after a friend, also a long-term cannabis smoker, switched to using medical cannabis from a doctor with dramatically better results for his chronic pain without feeling high or impaired.

This is a common story, because most black market cannabis contains high or very high THC and very little CBD. This matters when it comes to anxiety, because THC has what's called a biphasic effect: at small doses for most people it is good for anxiety, especially when using a strain with plenty of CBD in it. However, at higher doses, it can have the opposite effect and actually cause anxiety after an initial period of relieving it.

So someone may smoke or vape a high-THC cannabis flower and initially feel less anxious, but an hour or two later they may feel worse than before. Because the anxiety reaction doesn't happen immediately after they inhale it, it's common that this pattern is not discovered, and then they use even more THC in an attempt to stop the anxiety again. It leads to a roller coaster of mood and anxiety levels and is often quite confusing and stressful. It also doesn't happen to everyone at the same dose and THC amounts so two people could have the same amount of THC and have a different response.

If the black market cannabis they managed to get hold of is higher in CBD and lower in THC, they might smoke or vape the same amount and just get the anxiety relief without the later rebound anxiety, so it can be a total guessing game every time, which in itself causes more anxiety in a vicious cycle!

After I explained this to Dan, and once he overcame his initial scepticism that 'less is more' when it comes to THC for anxiety, he was excited to try some different strains. We chose a strain high in CBD and lower in THC for vaping, and added in a base of high-CBD, very low-THC oil to help calm the nervous system all day, rather than relying on the vaping when anxiety levels were already spiralling. This worked quite well and he was able to self-titrate successfully with no more rebound anxiety, increasing his general sense of calm and getting much better mental clarity.

He also had trouble falling asleep, taking up to two hours when 10–15 minutes or less is normal. But he had no problems staying asleep once he'd dropped off, so we introduced a so-called indica-dominant high-myrcene calming strain to vaporise before bedtime as part of an evening wind-down routine using my circadian rhythm reset protocol. This involves a gentle guided meditation recording, wearing blue-light-blocking glasses, coming off screens and avoiding caffeine, stimulants and eating late at night.

With all of my patients, cannabis and especially CBD can be a great catalyst and tool when used properly, but it's not a magic bullet cure-all. It's best combined with other holistic approaches to get the most control and relief in the long run – one piece of the bigger picture.

The evidence for anxiety

According to multiple studies and large data reviews as well as clinical evidence working with real patients, CBD has what we classify as 'good to strong' evidence for helping with anxiety. In fact, mental health uses for CBD and cannabis are some of the most well-researched indications. The anti-anxiety effects of CBD appear to come from many pathways in the brain, and one of them seems to affect our happy hormone serotonin.[6]

There are now many human research studies on the beneficial effects of cannabis, especially CBD, for anxiety conditions, including one that found CBD worked as well as the most common anti-anxiety prescription drugs for severe stress-induced anxiety, with fewer side effects.[7] A 2017 review of studies showed that CBD has clear anti-panic effects[8] in humans, and another review found that not only is it an effective anti-anxiety substance but it can also help buffer against THC side effects.[9, 10] A 2019 study found CBD to be effective for anxiety, sleep disruption and poor sleep quality in most patients, with only very rare and mild side effects in a few, which is well above the effectiveness for the best drug treatments, with much lower side effects. If those results were from a newly invented pharmaceutical drug, it would be branded a miracle drug![11]

Dozens more studies exist in animal models, since that was all scientists could study until recently, due to the restrictions on human cannabis and CBD as a 'class 1 drug of no medical value'. Thankfully, since the CBD and cannabis revolution over the past few years, research is fast increasing with each passing month.

PTSD

PTSD, or post-traumatic stress disorder, occurs after a trauma and is a separate diagnosis to anxiety. However, it can also be thought of as a very severe form of anxiety, where the brain loses its ability to return to a calm baseline state because the fear, stress and arousal circuits get triggered and won't turn off. PTSD happens when the trauma experience essentially gets stuck in the brain. Although experiencing some form of traumatic event is quite common, with more than two thirds of the general population undergoing a significant trauma at some point in their life,[12] not everyone who experiences trauma will get PTSD. After a trauma such as a natural disaster, an accident or an assault (either experienced yourself or bearing witness to such an event), it is normal to feel scared, sad, anxious and disconnected. But if those feelings don't fade and the sense of danger increases instead of improving, and if you begin to experience flashbacks and nightmares, reliving the trauma over and over, that is a sign you may be experiencing PTSD.

Whether or not someone develops PTSD from a trauma experience depends on how the brain processes the trauma, and also the nature of the trauma itself. If the trauma involves a threat to your life or personal safety, or is severe or prolonged, the risk of PTSD goes up, as this tends to create more severe stress on the brain's ability to process events and return to a normal baseline after a few weeks. Instead PTSD sufferers get stuck with a 24/7 sense of danger and threat that they cannot control or rationalise away. Other risk factors that increase the likelihood of the brain getting stuck in trauma include the trauma being unexpected and inescapable, with no control over what was happening; personal factors such as previous traumatic experiences (especially in childhood); family history of PTSD, depression, anxiety or other mental illness; history of substance abuse, or history of physical or sexual abuse. If you suspect you may have PTSD, which can sometimes go on undetected for years in milder forms, I urge you to get help from an experienced trauma counsellor, psychologist or doctor who is qualified in this area.

In my medical practice, seeing patients for cannabis medicine, I often worked with psychiatrists who would refer me patients with PTSD. We would add cannabis very carefully to help with their sleep disruption and nightmares, so they could get more traction with their other recovery therapies. Many times these patients had previously resorted to drinking alcohol before sleep to reduce the nightmares and flashbacks. They were using it as a form of self-medication, which was partly effective as alcohol decreases REM dreaming sleep, where the nightmares occur. Their drinking went down dramatically once we introduced a small dose of a high-THC, 'indica oil' before bedtime.

Most of the patients with PTSD who came to see me for cannabis had never tried it before. Many of them were police officers and veterans from the armed forces, so cannabis was a very big leap of faith for them after being told their whole careers to avoid using it! Cannabis and other psychoactive plant medicines, including psilocybin from specific types of mushrooms, are being increasingly studied and used successfully under psychotherapy guidance to help people recover from PTSD and trauma. There are no Western medicine drugs yet invented that can do this. We have a lot to learn from these plants as they become legal for medical use and more mainstream. This is something I am currently involved with from an academic perspective because I have seen first-hand the incredible effects cannabis can have when used properly.

Cannabis for PTSD

I have found high CBD medical cannabis useful clinically in helping with PTSD symptoms. This is supported by the preliminary research evidence, which suggests it helps with both daytime and night-time symptoms.[13] THC oil or capsules taken under medical supervision before bedtime may help dampen the fear response in the brain to help with nightmares and flashbacks, and can also help with insomnia. Because of the biphasic effect of THC on anxiety, THC-containing medical cannabis should be used only under the supervision of a doctor to ensure it helps not harms.

For additional information, see references[14, 15, 16, 17, 18, 19, 20].

How to use CBD wellness products (hemp CBD) for anxiety

- Try a full-spectrum or broad-spectrum CBD oil.
- Look for calming terpenes:
  - linalool – smells flowery, like lavender
  - myrcene – smells earthy/peppery, like hops, and is one of the most common terpenes
  - terpinolene – smells fresh, like a mix of flowers and pine
  - D-limonene – smells like lemons and has both anti-anxiety and antidepressant effects, so is thought of as a mood-balancing terpene.

Starting dose and titrating up

Try 10 mg of CBD first thing in the morning, at midday/early afternoon (12–2 p.m.) and at dinner time for a total of 30 mg/day. Stay at this dose for 1–2 weeks and test how you feel:

- Is the anxiety level improving?
- Is it still bad at a certain time of day (e.g. worse in the evening)?
- Are you still having trouble getting to sleep or staying asleep?

Score your anxiety level each day in the morning, afternoon and evening (after dinner) on a scale from 0–10, where 0 = no anxiety, 10 = unbearable/worst anxiety imaginable, and write down the results in your symptom tracker.

Slowly keep increasing the dose each week until anxiety is improving. After 1–2 weeks at the initial dose, try increasing one of the daily doses by 5 mg, depending on when your anxiety is worst, so for example if it gets worse in the late afternoon or evening, increase the midday dose, while if winding the mind down to prepare for bed is still an issue, increase the dinner dose.

If you reach 60 mg total per day of CBD, stay at this level for another 4–6 weeks before increasing again (since the effects of CBD can take weeks in some people, this will avoid increasing the dose unnecessarily).

Remember: there is no specific perfect dose that works for everyone when it comes to anxiety. Each person's endocannabinoid system balance is unique, so self-titration is the name of the game.

For maintenance: non-cannabis helpers to add

Once you reach a dose of CBD that is helping you, you can start adding in other anxiety-busters to help get even better effects and start to really rewire the brain anxiety pathways in the longer term:

- An anti-anxiety meditation. I recommend exploring a few simple meditation techniques to see which one resonates with you. Then practise it starting with just 5 minutes each day and adding a minute every few days until you reach 20 minutes, an amount most people can reasonably fit in.
- Calming herbs such as hops, valerian root, skullcap, chamomile.
- Swap coffee for herbal tulsi (also called holy basil) tea for a more natural energy without making anxiety worse with caffeine.
- Calming natural supplements such as L-theanine, inositol.
- An evening ritual after dinner to wind down the nervous system. This may include gentle calming music, dimming the lights, practising relaxing breathing or gentle stretching/yoga and getting off screens and social media.
- A wake-up-calm routine for the first minutes of the day. This may include avoiding checking emails and social media as soon as you wake up, a two-minute mindful breathing mini practice, and leaving time for a healthy breakfast with calming, nourishing GABA-supporting ingredients.

How to use medical cannabis products for anxiety

Only try this under the supervision of a doctor and, of course, if medical cannabis (containing THC) is legal where you live.

- Start with a high-CBD cannabis oil as your base for the daytime.

A strain high in CBD and very low in THC is the best starting
product for anxiety, taken by mouth.

- Look for calming terpenes for anxiety.
- Start with 5 mg three times a day: first thing in the morning,
  midday/early afternoon (12–2 p.m.) and dinner time, for a total of
  15 mg/day. Note: this is less than the dose for the CBD wellness
  products because medical cannabis oils have a bit more THC
  than hemp CBD does. This often means they work better at
  lower doses, due to the THC micro-dosing.
- Stay at this dose for a few days to one week and track your
  symptoms carefully.
- After this initial period, try increasing one of the daily doses by 5
  mg, depending on when your anxiety is worst, so for example if it
  gets worse in the late afternoon or evening, increase the midday
  dose, while if winding the mind down to prepare for bed is still
  an issue, increase the dinner dose.
- Because there is also a small amount of THC in these oils, slowly
  titrate the dose up by a few mg each week as needed to get
  relief from anxiety.
- When you reach 30 mg total per day of CBD (which will also
  include a small dose of THC if your medical cannabis oil contains
  0.5% or higher THC), stay at this dose for another 4–6 weeks
  before increasing the dose again, based on how you feel
  (everyone is a bit different).
- If you still don't see much improvement in anxiety after this
  period, slowly increase the dose again each week.
- In addition to medical cannabis, you can also try adding a hemp
  CBD oil or long acting hemp CBD product without THC, such
  as in a transdermal patch, to give a background of more CBD
  without adding additional THC from increasing the dose of the
  medical cannabis oil.

How to use vaporising cannabis flowers for anxiety

Vaporised cannabis can be used as an add-on to oils, either cannabis oils or hemp CBD oils.

Start with high-CBD, low-THC flowers, which are useful for helping to stop acute anxiety and panic attacks that may come on suddenly. This is the best way to start if you have never had THC before.

Just like with oils, start with high-CBD, low-THC flower. Strains of cannabis with high CBD to THC, around 20:1, include:

- Avidekel. This is approximately 15–18% CBD, 0.8–1% THC.
- ACDC. This is a very high-CBD, low-THC strain, up to 20% CBD and around 1% or less THC (average CBD to THC ratio is 24:1).
- Any CBD cultivar. Technically, any strain of cannabis can be bred into a high-CBD strain, including strains that were originally higher in THC – they breed out a large amount of the THC. There is no standard term for these high-CBD strains, but they are known by labels such as CBD cultivars or CBD flowers (when it's a dried cannabis product).
- If this has no effect, you can try a strain with more THC, known as a balanced strain, with equal amounts of CBD and THC.
- Start with a matchstick-head-sized amount, especially if it is a strain with more THC.
- For general anxiety and stress, vaporising CBD flower is a safe and effective way to take the edge off instead of having a glass of wine, for example.
- Cannabis flower can be used as a replacement for anxiety pills to help wean you off benzodiazepine (under medical supervision by your doctor).
- Can also be vaporised before doing a meditation or relaxation practice to help get the mind calm enough.
- Can be used before bedtime to help you get to sleep more easily and to wind down a busy mind, using a traditionally labelled indica or broad-leaf strain high in myrcene (see Chapter Eleven).

For additional information, see references [21, 22, 23, 24, 25, 26].

CHAPTER TEN

DEALING WITH LOW MOOD AND DEPRESSION

Cannabis's re-emergence as a modern plant medicine comes at a time of growing recognition and awareness of the importance of mental health. Increasingly we understand mental health as a gradient, not a binary state of perfectly well versus mentally ill. Especially with my parents' generation, people were perceived to be either fine and normal or having a mental breakdown, with no in-between. Mental health was just not discussed and was extremely stigmatised.

Before I began prescribing cannabis, I had already built a reputation as an integrative medicine doctor and developed a following of patients who were interested in a more holistic, less drug-focused approach to mental health. This meant mental health became a big part of my medical practice and area of expertise over the years, including treating patients for depression and low mood as well as anxiety, insomnia, stress-related disorders and burnout. These disorders are all related and sometimes difficult to tease apart in the real world. More often than not, my patients suffered from more than one at the same time. However, for the purposes of this book I have split them up in order to provide the most usable guide, and this chapter will focus mainly on depression and mood balance, while also touching on bipolar disorder.

In the treatment of complex mental health challenges and multiple diagnoses, I would often prescribe mindfulness and breathing techniques alongside medications and supplements. However, it became obvious that patients in a depressed state often didn't have the brain motivation or mental resources to stick with a technique long enough to reap the benefits. I realised that they needed a quicker win to get to a point where mindfulness and breathwork might help them.

What I discovered when it came to using other non-drug approaches in mental health, and especially in depression, was that it was not down to a patient's mental discipline or a need for them to just try harder. If you suffer from a mix of anxiety and depression or other mental health challenges, even if you want to meditate, or exercise, or engage with cognitive behavioural therapy, it's as if there's a brain roadblock in the way.

It's with these roadblocks that I have found cannabis to be very useful, providing a way to get that initial momentum for change that may have eluded patients for their entire lives.

When I started to use cannabis medicine and CBD to give patients that quick win, they were gradually able to stick with the more subtle and slower-acting non-drug therapies like mind-body practices, meditation and exercise. Because they were finally getting relief, their mental bandwidth naturally increased, as did their belief that it was possible to get better. That can be pretty life-changing after years of fighting an uphill battle and feeling that they'd already tried everything. Not to mention doing wonders for their self-esteem and self-belief, which had taken a beating after years of failed attempts to achieve the things they desperately wanted to.

I always say cannabis is not a magic bullet (nothing is!), but many of my patients would say it's the closest thing they have found to it. After trying every pharmaceutical drug available, cannabis is often the first thing that has helped them manage their symptoms without horrendous side effects, giving them that initial momentum to get their lives back on track.

One thing that really bothers me when doctors talk about the 'dangers' of medical cannabis is their focus on euphoria as a side effect. THC-containing cannabis may indeed produce a mood-lifting effect in many people with depression. However, as long as they are not overusing THC and also using CBD, and do not have a history of psychosis or mania (two areas where I tend to avoid THC altogether in my own practice), I really don't see a bit of euphoria as a side effect to be scared of. In fact, many people who suffer with chronic depression, and those with more mild cases of a disturbed chronic low mood, may actually have an endocannabinoid system that has become dysfunctional at balancing mood. A small dose of THC combined with CBD may be helping them to normalise ECS function, not make it worse. Someone who has never experienced depression, on the other hand, may find that THC may not do much for them in terms of mood elevation (I am one of those people).

Depression and mood balance

Depression, whether it's mild blues or a full-blown major depressive disorder, is a very common issue. Despite this, many people still suffer in silence due to the stigma around it. Here in the UK, where I live now, mental health in general and depression in particular is rarely a topic to be talked about openly. Although things are beginning to change, often the only time the subjects are discussed is when someone has what is referred to in hushed tones as a breakdown out of nowhere after seeming fine. Many of my nearest and dearest have suffered with depression, so I know first-hand how debilitating it can be and how often well-meaning advice can do more harm than good.

The integrative medicine view of depression

I've treated thousands of patients for depression over a decade in my practice using an integrative approach. Even as an intern and junior doctor in medical school it seemed clear to me that depression was not purely an SSRI deficiency, which meant it was not so easily solved by the wonder drug doctors hoped Prozac would be when it first came out. Depression is way more complicated and multifactorial than that, and all depressions are different. That is why there is not a single magic bullet that will cure everyone. The reason for this is that depression is like ADHD or chronic fatigue – it's a final common endpoint that has different triggers and contributing factors for each person. For some people, it can be as a result of early childhood trauma. For another, leaky gut is a major factor, or it can result from a series of losses or even a head injury. Often it's a combination of many factors that results in the brain getting stuck with the brakes on, as I like to say. When the brain feels under threat, it goes into protect-and-withdraw mode, which decreases activation in the left frontal lobe, leading to the symptoms so familiar to anyone who has experienced depression in some shape or form:

- trouble getting motivated
- social withdrawal
- negative thinking spirals
- feelings of being overwhelmed relating to decision-making, leading to doing nothing as the default
- appetite changes – sometimes craving carbs or alternatively having no appetite at all
- low energy
- sluggish thinking
- not being able to take pleasure or joy from your passions, hobbies or just life generally

One theory is that these are signs the brain does not feel safe and is trying to conserve energy because it feels there may be a threat: a form of brain self-protection if you will. The reasons for why someone gets depressed in the first place are manifold. Often significant stressors are involved in the lead-up to an initial episode. In recurrent depression, vulnerability to repeats seems to increase due to a brain-driven process called kindling. This means that the brain becomes more rigid and stuck and less able to break free of depression brain networks or adapt and change. Depression also involves a decrease in deep slow-wave restorative sleep.[1]

How cannabis and CBD can help with depression

When used properly, cannabis can help with multiple aspects of depression, including low energy, stress and anxiety and sleep. As always, cannabis is not a cure for depression but is a tool that should be used in the context of a wider holistic approach alongside lifestyle changes, working on the brain–gut connection and much more. However, a number of preliminary studies are beginning to uncover the mystery of how cannabis helps the depressed brain regain balance and become more flexible. For example, when depressed, the brain starts to make less of a chemical called brain-derived neurotrophic factor (BDNF). This is bad, because BDNF is the superhero chemical that promotes new brain cells and new learning in the brain – what is called neurogenesis. BDNF is like a brain anti-ageing chemical. When levels fall, the brain becomes less flexible in adapting to change, which means depression can become entrenched and harder to break out of (which may explain the kindling effect mentioned above).

We now think BDNF release is connected to healthy endocannabinoid system function,[2] which means that when the endocannabinoid system becomes dysfunctional, this may be a factor that messes with BDNF, and vice versa. Studies in mice have shown that CBD reduces neuroinflammation and improves neurogenesis (i.e. more BDNF!),[3] two critical factors that fight depression in the brain. We also have multiple animal studies where CBD works as a fast-acting antidepressant and is an effective treatment for depressed animals. In addition to working on depression, CBD also reduces aggressive behaviour in mice.

Although we are still some way from understanding exactly how the ECS regulates mood, preliminary studies have shown that it is critical to mood balance and emotional regulation; and we know that dysregulation of the ECS is involved in the three major mental health disorder areas – anxiety disorders, depression disorders and schizophrenia/psychotic disorders. So far, CBD hemp products on their own have not been tested in formal research trials in humans for depression.

For additional information, see references[4, 5, 6, 7, 8, 9].

Bipolar depression and schizophrenia: risks of cannabis use

One of the most common questions I am asked by my patients and my medical colleagues is: what about cannabis causing psychosis or mania?

The relationship between cannabis use and psychosis, schizophrenia and bipolar mania is complex. One of the complicating factors is that the cannabis type in the published studies on these disorders is high-THC street cannabis without much, if any, CBD. And the studies rely on data from recreational cannabis users, not medical cannabis patients. The use of cannabis in those users was unsupervised, recreational and smoked. This is in total contrast to how I use cannabis as a doctor: supervised, careful medical use with mainly high-CBD, low-THC products and oral dosing (i.e. longer acting) as the base of therapy. To compare the two is like comparing apples with oranges. In my clinical practice prescribing medical cannabis to patients, including those with anxiety disorders and depression, I have never had a single case of psychosis or mania after starting medical cannabis. However, I do not use products containing significant THC for any patient who has a personal history (including a first-degree relative) of psychosis, schizophrenia, schizoaffective disorder or bipolar manic episodes. For these patients, I would recommend high-CBD, very low-THC products only under close monitoring by a physician and while working alongside their psychiatrist. This may include hemp-based CBD wellness products, since they definitely have only trace THC.

It is important not to dismiss the possibility that cannabis use increases the risk of psychosis in genetically vulnerable individuals, as there does seem to be a risk, although a small one, from the research we have so far. But it's also important to emphasise that the risk seems to be the THC, not hemp-based CBD products. In one study, for example, high-THC smoked street cannabis use and cannabis-induced psychosis increased the risk of conversion to schizophrenia, and younger users seemed to have a higher conversion rate. Another theory based on the current studies available suggests that high-THC, low-CBD recreational cannabis use can dispose a vulnerable subgroup in the population to schizophrenia,[10] or perhaps speed up the unmasking of the disease (meaning they already have it, but it may be triggered or show up sooner).[11] Based on the research so far, there also appears to be a dose–response relationship (i.e. a connection)[12] between the smoking of high-THC cannabis and the risk of schizophrenia, especially in genetically vulnerable young people.[13] The only types of cannabis included in these studies were very high-THC, low-CBD cultivars, which are rarely used medically in large doses and certainly not as the main base of therapy for mental health conditions.

There are, however, other studies done in people who already have schizophrenia or bipolar that have found a positive association between black-market high-THC cannabis use and attenuated reductions in grey matter density,[14] meaning that those who smoked cannabis had less grey matter brain shrinkage on brain scanning (using fMRI imaging). What this means in plain English is that it possibly made their brains work better, not worse, which is contrary to popular belief and also many other studies. It was only an association, not a cause relationship, however, so we need more studies to investigate it further to say for sure what it may mean. Another study found that adolescent (teen and pre-teen) recreational cannabis use was associated with better cognitive function in schizophrenia but not in bipolar[15] – so again each brain disorder may be different in how it responds to cannabis, as well as the type of cannabis, the amount of CBD and THC and other contaminants.

My friend and colleague, psychiatrist and researcher Dr Lili Galindo, has spent the last seven years studying the relationship between cannabis and schizophrenia, and her latest findings are just starting to be published.[16] They shed some light on why some people may experience paranoia or other negative mood effects from THC in cannabis; it may be down to them having a different type of CB1 receptor variant that links onto a specific type of serotonin receptor. This special receptor duo is called a CB1-5HT2A heteromer. Those who make more of them may be the same people who are at increased vulnerability or risk of developing or triggering the onset of a brain psychosis disorder such as schizophrenia when they use THC, especially regularly, at higher amounts and at younger ages, before the brain is fully developed. In her most recent study, Dr Lili and her team are finding preliminary evidence that cannabis may actually help the thinking impairment from the drug side effects used to treat schizophrenia, meaning for some people with schizophrenia, cannabis with THC make actually alleviate some of their symptoms and medication side effects and improve their quality of life. This is a ground-breaking concept in mental health and medical cannabis.

What we do know quite a lot about already, however, is that CBD seems to have antipsychotic (meaning protects from psychosis) brain effects through a number of different pathways:

- In a 2018 study, researchers looked at the effects of CBD on different brain areas in people at high risk of psychosis. The participants received a single oral dose of 600 mg of CBD and then underwent brain imaging while they did a verbal learning task. The results showed that CBD can normalise brain function in the specific brain regions implicated in psychosis.
- In another study, a drug for psychosis called amisulpride was compared to CBD as a treatment in acute schizophrenia.[17] Both CBD and the drug treatment led to clinical improvement, but CBD had far fewer side effects. Interestingly, the CBD also showed an increase in the brain's natural endocannabinoid anandamide. This change in anandamide level was significantly associated with clinical improvement.
- In a small group of healthy people, pre-treatment with CBD prevented the acute psychotic symptoms of a large dose of THC. This study also showed that CBD had an opposite effect on brain function to THC based on fMRI brain imaging.
- A 2015 systematic review of CBD published in the journal *Schizophrenia Research* showed that CBD has the ability to

counteract psychotic symptoms and cognitive impairment associated with THC-containing cannabis use.[18] In addition, CBD may lower the risk of developing psychosis related to (high-THC) cannabis use.

So, in conclusion, it seems that CBD may be helpful in treating psychosis in schizophrenia, bipolar and other related disorders and can help buffer the effects of THC. It further appears that some people may be more genetically at risk to the negative effects of THC on mood or in triggering psychosis, although the risk generally is still very low. Even if CBD is not enough on its own, it may be useful in combination with drug therapy to reduce the need for high doses of the more potent antipsychotic drugs, which have many side effects. Studies suggest properly prescribed cannabis may improve both brain function and quality of life in patients with these types of brain disorders, which are very difficult to treat and extremely disabling.

My introduction to the counterculture movement

After medical school, with my doctorate in hand, and before starting my residency, which is your first junior doctor job before going into private practice, I decided to go travelling in Asia for three months. I went without a plan; just a backpack and a Lonely Planet guide and also some word-of-mouth recommendations from other backpackers on places to check out that were still off the grid.

I ended up at an alternative yoga retreat on a beach in Thailand and found myself at the heart of a counterculture movement where people had traded 9–5 jobs for living in simple thatched huts, spending their days doing yoga and meditation and creating art of some sort ... as well as taking LSD on Tuesday mornings! In this highly creative community of Westerners who had opted out of mainstream 9–5 work culture, cannabis, for many of them, was a central part of the culture, far more so than alcohol; in fact many of them didn't drink at all.

The cannabis in Thailand was grown in the jungle without any fertiliser and didn't make people super-stoned. However, many people swore by it for helping them balance their mood and enhance their creativity, considering it the best medicine to help with chronic depression, a very common ailment among the community. Some of them told me that using cannabis had helped them give up alcohol. Alcohol was what some had been using previously to self-medicate symptoms of depression, with significantly worse side effects, including addiction.

These people were hippies, not scientists, but I was intrigued by their stories, and the same theme kept popping up with dozens of people I met over those months of hanging out by my little beach hut. It got me reconsidering my own beliefs about cannabis being universally bad for mood and depression. And I had to wonder why alcohol was a socially acceptable and legal intoxicant despite its known negative effects on the brain, especially a brain suffering with depression.

As a scientist, I found it intriguing that this Thai jungle weed seemed to be quite different from the heavy stoner weed I had seen smoked in Canada as a teen and which often left people sleepy and couch-locked, even though it was the same plant.

Years later, after I started to use cannabis as a medicine, I realised that the local Thai jungle weed, known as kancha, was a lower-THC variety of cannabis, higher in CBD and more of what was traditionally labelled a sativa-dominant strain. It was a very different plant to the typical very high-THC traditionally labelled indica cannabis most people had access to back in Canada at the time.

Interestingly, just as in India, the cannabis plant was used for hundreds of years in Thailand as a textile and as a medicine before its ban in 1934. It is likely that it came into Thailand from India, with local varieties shifting and adapting over time due to the differences in climate and humidity. The very high humidity in Thailand was probably one of the factors that led to the unique strains of cannabis seen on the beach, as the plant had to make slightly different chemicals to fight off moulds and adapt to the climate.

The bong alarm clock

Long before I was adding cannabis to my medical practice, I had friends who used it on their own to manage their mental health. I was initially very sceptical about the claims they were making, still believing, like most doctors and the public, that cannabis was a harmful illegal drug of no medicinal value. I also feared it would make their mental health worse, especially when it came to issues like depression.

When I was first starting out in my medical practice, I had a month where I was in-between apartments and needed a room to rent. I was still in debt from medical school, my boyfriend was away and I didn't want to sleep in a hotel by myself for a month (these were the days before Airbnb!), so Chloe, a friend from university, offered me a spare room in a large house share outside the city, where a collection of artists, film-makers, musicians and creatives lived.

They grew their own vegetables, and even a few cannabis plants, which one of the roommates used to make topical balms for period pains for friends. She would dry the plants by hanging them from the rafters in her bedroom, filling the house with a pleasant aroma.

The room I was renting was in the basement, and I will never forget my first morning there. As I lay in bed trying to catch a few more minutes' sleep, I became aware of a loud gurgling sound. I thought maybe it was a problem with the pipes, then looked up to see Chloe sitting at the end of the bed taking a massive hit on a bong pipe! 'Morning!' she said cheerily, handing me a cup of green tea.

This bong alarm clock became a strange but fun morning ritual during my time there. My spare room apparently was where the weed was stashed, and Chloe used some every morning to activate and manage her mood. She had been diagnosed with many things in the past by various doctors, including something called borderline personality disorder and depression, which she had tried to manage conventionally with medications, but had not found the pills all that helpful after giving them a fair shot. Instead she had settled on her own solution: a small amount of cannabis vaporised (in the water bong) and via an oral oil, along with a strict healthy diet, sleep and exercise routine that seemed to work quite well and kept her level of function high without any side effects. She had a successful career and social life and felt that using cannabis to medicate was part of this success. We now know that borderline personality disorder, despite the sensationalist name, is probably nothing to do with personality but is in fact a neuroendocrine disorder involving malfunctioning stress response systems and serotonin disturbances,[19] which may explain why cannabinoids can help.

At the time I thought it was just an excuse to get high each morning before work, but I have since successfully treated hundreds of patients with depression and mood disorders with medical cannabis, and many of my patients with similar symptoms find using a vaporiser first thing in the morning an incredibly effective way to activate it immediately, as oils take longer to work. It has allowed some of them to actually get to work on time and dramatically reduce their sick days. Using a low-THC variety means they don't feel impaired, just normal, and in fact for some people a certain amount of THC seems to be an important factor in making it work well for their mood management.

Bong alarm clocks, however, are decidedly not Dr Dani-approved!

How to use CBD wellness products (hemp CBD) for mood management

- CBD oil alone is not a proven treatment for depression, but because depression and anxiety often overlap, CBD can definitely help with the anxiety component as a start. CBD seems to work as an antidepressant in animals, but we don't yet have human studies on CBD only for this purpose. In my clinical experience, I used a low-THC medical cannabis product (but still with more THC than hemp) as a starting point, and for some people even adding a bit more THC (along with CBD) was very useful when the right strain was picked.
- Use a full-spectrum or broad-spectrum CBD oil.

- Look for uplifting, mood-balancing terpenes:
  - D-limonene – smells like lemons and has both anti-anxiety and antidepressant effects so it can be thought of as a mood-balancing terpene
  - alpha-pinene
  - beta-caryophyllene

Starting dose and titrating up

Take 10 mg of CBD first thing in the morning, at midday/early after-noon (12–2 p.m.) and at dinner time, for a total of 30 mg/day. Stay at this dose for a few days to a week and track your symptoms carefully to test how you feel:

- Is your mood improving?
- Is it still bad at a certain time of day (e.g. worse in the evening)?
- Are you having trouble getting to sleep or staying asleep? If so, you may benefit from sleep support – see Chapter Eleven.

Score your mood and energy level each day, in the morning, after-noon and evening (after dinner) on a scale from 0–10, where 0 = no motivation/severe low mood, 10 = motivated, happy and content, and write down the results in your symptom tracker

You can slowly keep increasing the dose each week. If you reach 60 mg total per day of CBD, stay here for another 4–6 weeks before increasing again (since the effects of CBD may take weeks or even months to fully kick in, this will avoid increasing the dose unnecessarily).

Remember: there is no specific perfect dose that works for every-one exactly the same. Each person's endocannabinoid system bal-ance is unique, so self-titration is the name of the game. Hemp CBD may not work for everyone with depression. It seems to help some, while in others it does not appear to have much of an effect and may also be dose-dependant. So it's best to work with a health practition-er who understands cannabis, as well as exploring other treatments for depression both natural and conventional.

If you have been diagnosed with bipolar, CBD may help reduce side effects of the other medications people need to take daily to treat the disorder, according to some case reports (no large studies available) but always consult your doctor before trying any new supplement, even CBD, to err on the side of caution. It is also extra important that in such a case, the CBD product that is used is from a company that tests their products and has a certificate of analysis (see Chapter Five) to ensure it is not contaminated with THC, since this can be dangerous (especially when not done under special supervision) if you suffer with manic episodes or psychosis (also see Chapter Six for cautions and caveats).

Non-cannabis helpers for depression and low mood

In addition to medical cannabis, I use other natural approaches like supplements, botanicals and mind-body approaches that can help with depression and chronic low moods:

- Compassion or loving-kindness meditation. This type of meditation wakes up the left frontal lobe, which becomes depressed or sluggish in depression. Many guided versions can be found online, and I make a recorded version for my clients to help them do it.
- 20 minutes of cardio exercise most days of the week. This has been proven to raise serotonin levels, boost endorphins and natural endocannabinoids and also increase BDNF (brain-derived neurotrophic factor) and decrease cortisol stress hormones.
- Fish-derived omega-3 fatty acid supplement. Depression has an inflammatory component and EPA fatty acids from fish may help over time at doses between 1 and 4 g/day.
- Zinc. Can be tried alongside natural therapies or also added to an SSRI drug to make it work better at lower doses. Dose: 20–30 mg/day.
- B vitamins and folic acid. These are needed to help make healthy mood neurotransmitters, and borderline B12 or other B

vitamin deficiencies as well as folate deficiencies are common in depressed adults. Dose: B complex 100 mg/day; folic acid 1 mg/ day in a supplement.

- Vitamin D. 10,000 IU/week may benefit mood, especially because borderline or low vitamin D levels can cause depression. This is an under-treated problem in countries far from the equator like the UK, Canada and many parts of the US.

- St John's wort. This herb works for some people with mild to moderate depression (similar efficacy to an SSRI drug in some studies), but only when the product is high-quality, properly extracted and standardised. This is also not a good botanical medicine for patients on many other medications, since it has so many possible drug interactions, but so far no issue has been seen combining with low-THC, high-CBD medical cannabis clinically speaking, but no large formal research studies have yet studied this possible combination.

> Hemp CBD oils and medical cannabis oils high in CBD and low in THC should not be overly sedating. If they are making you feel tired, check the label to see if the product you are using is rich in myrcene, a terpene that can be too sedating for the daytime in some people, and also check the product is not labelled as an indica, even though technically most will be hybrids.

How to use medical cannabis products for depression

Only try this under the supervision of a doctor and, of course, if medical cannabis (containing THC) is legal where you live.

- Start with a high-CBD cannabis oil or capsule as your base. Choose a strain high in CBD and very low in THC.

- Take 5 mg of CBD first thing in the morning, 5 mg at midday/ early afternoon (12–2 p.m.) and 5 mg at dinner time, for a total of 15 mg/day. This is less than the dose for the CBD wellness products because medical cannabis oils have a bit more THC than hemp CBD does. This often makes it work better at lower doses, due to the THC micro-dosing.

- Increase the dose slowly using the 'start low, go slow' approach and under the supervision and advice of your prescribing doctor, since depression dosing is different for everyone and needs to be monitored as you go.
- If your sleep is disrupted, discuss with your doctor about sleep support and what may be right for you (see Chapter Eleven).
- If one product seems not to be working after a 4–6 week trial, choose another made from a different strain if possible (look for more uplifting terpenes, for example).

How to use vaporising cannabis flowers for low mood

- Especially if you are new to THC cannabis, start by trying a high-CBD, low-THC flower (CBD to THC ratio of 20:1) that may be labelled as sativa-dominant with low myrcene and rich in D-limonene terpenes for maximum pick-me-up potential.
- Start with a matchstick-head-sized amount, and take a single inhalation first thing in the morning if you have trouble with morning motivation, low mood and fatigue.
- If this has no effect, you can try the same technique with a new strain with more THC and similar terpenes, known as a balanced strain (i.e. with equal amounts of CBD and THC), but only if there are no contraindications, such as risk of mania or psychosis or history of schizophrenia or bipolar.

CHAPTER ELEVEN

IMPROVING SLEEP

Sleep used to be considered a basic human function that we just did naturally, and even took for granted. However, in the last few decades our sleep as a society has become massively dysfunctional, and increasingly medicalised. Recent data shows that around 16 million adults in the UK suffer from sleepless nights and a third suffer from actual insomnia.[1] Double that number have disrupted sleep, and the picture is similar across the Western world. Problems with sleep are not just night-time problems. Insomnia and disrupted sleep are very often the result of 24-hour nervous system hyperarousal and dysregulation. If we only treat the issue of poor sleep right before going to bed, we are unlikely to get to the bottom of the problem for good, no matter how many sleeping pills or supplements we take.

Part of the problem is that most of us who live in cities (and even many people who live in less urban areas) exist in what I like to call an 'anti-sleep environment'. Almost every aspect of modern culture works against the natural sleep-wake cycles of light vs darkness, sleep and rest. Our lives are set up to keep our brains constantly engaged and stimulated, well into the evenings after the sun has set. Instead of winding down at night as our ancestors did, we wind *up* – we sit in front of blue-light screens to watch TV, our phones or our computers, or we go out at night to socialise, consuming alcohol and caffeine to stay alert. Then we expect our nervous systems to be able to wind down instantly on demand the moment our heads hit the pillow. When, inevitably, this doesn't happen, we stress about getting to sleep because we know we have to wake up to a morning alarm feeling groggy, needing caffeine, and do it all over again. For many people, feeling tired during the day due to poor sleep is accepted as normal.

It is no surprise then that we are facing an insomnia and sleeping problem epidemic, which also causes a host of mental and physical health problems during the daytime. When I ask my patients and wellness clients at the first visit and in our group programmes, 'When was the last time you woke up naturally, feeling refreshed?' most people cannot remember. For those who do remember, it is often only on their last holiday that they experienced a truly refreshed start to the day. For many, even then good sleep eluded them.

What's the big deal? Why sleep matters

Getting into sleep debt from a chronic lack of non-restorative sleep seriously affects how your brain works, and can impinge on your brainpower, meaning your cognition and critical thinking. A bad sleep even for even one night impairs memory to a similar extent to being drunk. Sleep debt can even change the way the brain sees the world. For example, poor sleepers appear to be more sensitive to negative cues in the environment vs positive ones, possibly causing the brain to interpret the environment in a more bleak, threatening way.[2]

Disturbed sleep can even have a negative effect on your relationship with your partner. A study of over 1000 married people found that sleep disturbance was a signficant predictor of the health of the marriage, regardless of age or gender.[3] From a vanity perspective, sleep deprivation has been shown in multiple studies to contribute to weight gain.[4, 5] That stubborn fat around your middle that won't budge with exercise or diet may also be a result of the effects of disrupted cortisol (your stress hormone) due, in part, to poor sleep.[6] Even your skin suffers, as found in a study on sleep and skin ageing, where the poor sleepers had multiple increased signs of skin ageing when compared to the matched good sleepers.[7]

Letting go of something vs taking something for sleep

As an integrative medicine doctor who specialises in sleep and fatigue issues, I always say that restoring healthy sleep starts not with adding something (i.e. a pill or supplement) but with letting something go. If we want to sleep better, it is time to reconsider the screens we watch at night (and even in bed!), which disrupt sleep hormone production (melatonin) in the brain. We need to look at our relationship with the caffeine that fragments our sleep and makes us feel unrested in the morning; for some people who are ultra-sensitive to caffeine or have anxiety, even one or two coffees mid-morning can affect sleep that night. We have to question the glass of wine (or three!) that we drink to relax after a long day, which ultimately disrupts the restorative REM sleep that we need. And, crucially, we have to examine the absence of relaxation, meditation and a nervous system wind-down period in our evening routine.

But the reality is that in addition to these lifestyle shifts (which are not always easy to make), there are many people who also *do* need to take something to help restore their sleep patterns, or at least get them back on track and break the cycle of using uppers like caffeine to wake up in the morning and downers like alcohol to crash into sleep at night.

I had one patient, Doug, who was referred to me from his GP for insomnia. He claimed he had tried everything, including meditation, sleeping pills and melatonin. When we dug into his sleep history and habits in detail, however, I discovered he regularly had an energy drink just before lunch to perk him up. The other doctors he had seen had thought this caffeine source was too far away from his 11 p.m. bedtime to be affecting his sleep, but I had seen similar cases before of ultra-slow metabolisers of caffeine.

From an integrative medicine treatment approach for sleep, I get rid of any and all sources of caffeine for a period of six weeks in patients who have any issue with sleep. It took some convincing, but in the end, Doug agreed to cut it out completely for the trial period.

In addition, I gave him a very small dose of THC (2 mg) to add to his melatonin instead of his prescription sleeping pill if he still had problems sleeping after a week without caffeine. To stabilise his energy levels without resorting to energy drinks, we started a botanical supplement with cordyceps, lion's mane mushrooms and liquorice root.

Two weeks after getting rid of the caffeine completely, Doug had many nights where he only took the melatonin and didn't need cannabis at all, or his sleeping pill. On the days where he was still having trouble winding down at night, he used the micro dose of cannabis oil with THC in it, with good results. We also added CBD oil for during the day to help with his overall stress levels. Six months later, he was sleeping well most nights for the first time in many years, his daytime energy had improved and he even noticed an improvement in his memory and ability to focus at work.

The Western medicine approach to insomnia

The main tool most people are given when they go to their doctor with sleeping problems is some basic advice on sleep hygiene. This includes a variety of practices, such as establishing a regular bedtime routine, removing distractions from the bedroom, avoiding screens before bed and cutting out caffeine and alcohol in the evening as well as heavy meals. This may be effective for mild sleeping issues, but for many people, these changes are not enough to solve the problem. Alternatively, patients are given prescription sleeping pills, which is the sledgehammer approach to insomnia; it knocks us out immediately, while allowing us to continue with the rest of our sleep-damaging habits and environment.

In addition to prescription sleeping pills, many people rely on over-the-counter antihistamines to get to sleep, or a glass of wine with dinner. Unfortunately, both of these non-prescription 'sleep aids' actually disrupt the normal sleep architecture (patterns) and lead to poor-quality and fragmented sleep. This self-medication contributes to the vicious cycle of waking up feeling tired in the morning, followed by the dreaded 4 p.m. energy crash, and then more caffeine, stimulants, alcohol or other substances just to equalise our energy levels and get through the week.

When canna-sceptics (including other doctors) ask me about the evidence for cannabis and sleep, pointing to the fact that it is only preliminary as far as the published literature is concerned, I am quick to remind them that many sleeping pills routinely prescribed to patients, as well as over-the-counter sleep aids, have only been approved officially for short and medium term use, or are drugs used for sleep as an 'off-label' use, meaning the drug was originally made to treat a different condition, such as some antipsychotic drugs used for sleep. There remains a huge debate in the research as well as among doctors about how effective and risky long term daily sleeping pill use is, and it obviously also depends on which drug is used. Some studies report that for certain prescription sleeping pills, patients still self-report sleeping better even months after starting treatment and have acceptable side effect rates and that the harms have been overstated. Other human studies on prescription sleeping pills (classified as 'sedative-hypnotic drugs') have concluded that even occasional use of these drugs (fewer than 18 pills prescribed per year) is associated with a a threefold increased risk of death, as well as worse mental health outcomes, independent of other medical issues or conditions.[8, 9, 10, 11, 12, 13, 14]

Regardless, it has been my experience clinically over many years of treating thousands of people with trouble sleeping that these pills are often overprescribed and can do more harm than good or, in many cases, are not particulary effective without significant side effects when relied upon daily. That is still better than someone not sleeping at all however but when more natural methods can be tried, I think it is critical to try these first, or at least use them together with sleeping pills to reduce the doses needed, side effects and potential risks.

Cannabinoids used for sleep and for other related symptoms such as chronic pain and anxiety, do not appear to increase mortality risk, unlike some of the other sleeping pills. If anything, when used appropriately, they may even contribute to enhanced longevity due to their neuroprotective benefits, especially in older adults and people who have dysfunctional, underperforming or dysregulated endocannabinoid systems.

When taking something for sleep is needed

So as well as letting go of common modern life habits that disrupt sleep, sometimes it is necessary to consider taking something for sleep. Cannabis is one option, although by no means the silver bullet that will instantly restore perfect sleep forever. However, it can be used in low doses to help restore and support sleep that has become dysfunctional for reasons such as:

- chronic fatigue syndrome and the 'tired but wired' nervous system
- chronic pain keeping us awake
- anxiety and toxic stress preventing us from falling asleep
- treatment-resistant insomnia that has been failed by other approaches.

Before trying cannabis, I usually start with other low-risk botanical and supplement sleep support and non-pill approaches. However, most of the patients I see for sleep issues are already hooked on very strong prescription sleeping pills such as benzodiazepines, Ambien and zopiclone. In many cases they have tried, and failed, to come off their sleeping pills multiple times. Behavioural approaches such as CBT for sleep and non-cannabis herbal sleep aids are not always enough to get the sleep train back on track, and often people have had so many fails that improving sleep relatively quickly is pretty important. Especially when there are other chronic issues where cannabis may also help, low- to very-low-dose cannabis can be a good option, and one I have used in my practice successfully with many hundreds of patients.

The goal is not needing it every night once sleep is back on track. After an initial period (3–12 months) of taking it nightly, many of my patients now only use a tiny dose of cannabis oil 1–2 days a week.

In this period, in addition to cannabis, we work on the non-drug approaches to sleep, as well as adding safe 'sleepy herbs' such as passionflower, skullcap, valerian and hops that work well in synergy with low-dose cannabis.

My sleep protocol has become so popular and successful that I now begin all of my resilience and burnout recovery programmes with the seven-day circadian rhythm reset programme before we tackle any other issues, since sleep is the foundation for healthy stress response and lowering daytime anxiety as well as fatigue levels. So it's safe to say that cannabis is not the magic bullet for sleep that some may have hoped for, but it does provide another useful tool when used in moderation in the right context with the right product.

The one exception to not needing to take cannabis every night is sleep dysfunction alongside chronic pain. In these cases, where the cause of the chronic pain (such as degenerative conditions of the spine like spinal stenosis) is not curable, patients will often continue to use a small dose of night-time cannabis daily or almost daily in place of painkillers and sleeping pills, which they have found works better with less side effects for their pain and sleep.

The endocannabinoid system and sleep

Our endocannabinoid system has been found to modulate sleep and regulate the stability of the various sleep stages.[15] We know, for example, that blocking the CB1 receptor promotes wakefulness (i.e. decreases sleepiness).[16] THC, on the other hand, partially activates the CB1 receptor, which may enhance NREM sleep. NREM sleep is the dreamless sleep phase, including the deep-sleep phase we need where the brain and body repair cells, tissues and the immune system. We are still learning all the ways that the endocannabinoid system controls sleep cycles, and have only just scratched the surface so far.[17]

CBD vs THC for sleep

For some people, CBD on its own may actually promote wakefulness, while others report that a hemp-based CBD oil without THC helps them get to sleep and feel better in the morning. Why the difference? There are a number of possible reasons for the variation in responses. One reason may be the differences in each person's sleep-regulating endocannabinoid system, varying causes and types of sleeping issues, and also differences in the dose and product taken.

For example, if the sleep issue has to do with dreaming sleep (REM sleep), CBD may have a different effect than if it is more to do with non-dreaming sleep (NREM sleep). The picture may change again if the main sleep issue seems to be falling asleep only. The effect of CBD on sleep may also depend on how well rested someone is: in someone who is sleep-deprived, their ratio of REM to NREM stage 4 sleep changes to compensate for the sleep debt, and CBD may alter this. In plain English, what that means is that when you are sleep-deprived, the brain compensates by having more deep sleep and less dreaming sleep, which CBD seems to affect differently. There have been no studies using CBD on its own for comparing sleep-deprived vs well-rested people, so we still don't have a clear answer to the exact difference this makes.

The exact effect of CBD on its own without THC for sleep is still unclear from a research study perspective. THC is more well known and widely studied for its sleep-promoting effects, and this effect is helped again, it appears, by minor cannabinoids and calming, sedating terpenes like myrcene in certain strains, often labelled as 'indica'. In most cases if using medical cannabis for sleep, less is more. A small dose of THC can help with sleep, while too much can lead to a hangover feeling or morning grogginess and reduced short-term memory and energy the next day. These effects are more likely if you are new to THC – for experienced users, this grogginess may go away[18] – but it is still best to use the lowest effective dose. THC in high doses, it seems, can decrease REM sleep, which is the dreaming sleep believed to be important for memory consolidation (i.e. getting rid of stuff you don't need and keeping the information that is important after each day). That may be one reason why THC before bed helps those with PTSD to reduce their nightmares, which occur in the REM sleep stage. If you do not have PTSD, however, you don't want to lose out on REM sleep or disrupt the normal sleep cycles. It seems that very low doses (less than 10 mg) of THC do not affect REM sleep or the other sleep phases negatively.

Most of my patients who need THC for sleep use well below 10 mg/night unless there is a secondary reason such as severe treat-ment-resistant pain. In some people, too much THC over a long peri-od may cause more exhaustion, especially if not used alongside a hefty dose of CBD, which tends to buffer this effect (so caution is needed if someone already has a lot of daytime fatigue, such as with MS or chronic fatigue syndrome). Again, the name of the game with medical cannabis for sleep is that even though THC may be respon-sible for sleepier effects, using CBD with it to buffer the potential side effects is a good way to go, at least to start with. When CBD is used in combination with THC, it does not tend to make most people feel more awake (although occasionally it can!), but simply helps the THC work well with less chance of disrupting REM sleep.[19]

Steve's story

Steve came to see me to get help with using medical cannabis for his sleep, after his GP became concerned that he had been smoking street can-nabis as a sleep aid for years. When we went through his health history, Steve was overall quite healthy but had a stressful job with often long hours into the evening as a corporate lawyer. He travelled for work across time zones, which tended to disrupt his sleep further. He had been using a small amount of smoked cannabis a few days a week for many years to help him fall asleep. On further questioning, he had also tried a very potent high-THC cannabis oil from a non-medical dispensary since it was easier to travel with, but found it left him feeling groggy in the morning. When he didn't use cannabis, he had a glass of wine to help him unwind and fall asleep. Without cannabis, it often took him up to two hours to get to sleep, especially after a long day or with changing time zones. He *generally slept well once he fell asleep, but wine fragmented and disrupted his normal sleep cycles, making him feel unrested in the morning.*

We decided to try him on vaporised cannabis using a low dose flower (THC to CBD ratio of around 3:1) to eliminate or at least reduce to minimal the potential risk to the lungs of smoking. I also got him to start taking 3 mg of melatonin when he was crossing time zones or when his normal time for going to sleep was disrupted. The combination of low-dose vaporised cannabis when needed, plus the melatonin, worked beautifully without any daytime side effects. After a few months, he was also open to other non-drug approaches, including mindfulness meditation. He decided to take up this practice for 10 minutes a day, which over time he found helped shut off his work mind after a hectic day and further helped his sleep.

The published research on cannabis and sleep

The published research evidence on cannabinoids and sleep is often confusing and unclear. One of the reasons for this is that most of the bigger studies, at least in humans, have been done using synthetic THC cannabis drugs like nabilone. So using this drug version of THC on it's own rather than whole plant extract can impact results in a huge way, especially since THC without the other minor cannabinoids and terpenes which we think contribute to the entourage effect are removed. This leaves only the most potent psychoactive chemical THC all by itself in the pill, something that unsurprisingly from a botanical medicine perspective, tends to cause more side effects and be less effective, at least in my clinical experience with my many patients. Another issue is that many of those studies were set up to study factors other than sleep, so the sleep data was a by-product (in scientist-speak a 'secondary endpoint') rather than the main study purpose, which also can affect results.

Animal studies

In animal models such as rats, the effects of CBD on sleep have been mixed so far. One study found that CBD infused into the brain (in the area called the lateral hypothalamus)[20] suppressed sleep and increased alertness, but another study injected the same brain region and found that this led to an increase in a sleep-promoting brain chemical called adenosine. These two findings contradict each other. In other animal studies, the confusion theme is repeated: CBD especially at high doses promotes sleep, but in other studies it increases alertness and decreases sleep (REM sleep specifically).[21] Contradicting this, another rat study found that CBD improved the REM[22] disruption caused by anxiety. If this were found to be true in large studies in humans, it could mean that CBD might actually help to normalise sleep if the sleep problems were due to anxiety (or the extreme end of the spectrum, PTSD. Certainly in people with anxiety, there are countless reports of successful self-use of CBD oil to help with both anxiety and sleep, something I have noticed time and time again.

These confusing and often conflicting results from animal studies on CBD and sleep highlight how much we have yet to learn.

Human studies

In people with specific sleep problems, CBD may prove useful. For example, in a small study of four patients with Parkinson's disease, CBD reduced their REM sleep dysfunction associated with the disease, leading to improved sleep.[23] Another study looked at the effect of CBD on people with anxiety or poor sleep and found that sleep improved in two thirds of people and even more had a reduction in anxiety. So if your sleep issues are related to anxiety, CBD may have some benefit.[24] It may also be promising for REM sleep disorders (e.g. sleepwalking, acting out dreams) and for reducing daytime fatigue, but more studies are needed to support these preliminary findings.

Another study of 2000 people looked at the cannabis plant-derived pharmaceutical drug Sativex (which is a 1:1 ratio of CBD to THC) and found that it improved sleep in addition to their other symptoms.[25] Another study looked at the effects of CBD vs THC on sleep in healthy volunteers. It found that THC on its own was sedative (sleep-promoting), while CBD on its own had alerting properties, and the CBD counteracted the sedative effect of 15 mg THC when subjects were given both (THC followed directly by CBD).[26]

Other researchers have looked at isolated THC (not whole-extract cannabis oil with terpenes and other cannabinoids) for insomnia and found it helped them to get to sleep. However, higher doses (20–30 mg) led to a hangover feeling the next morning.[27] Isolated THC tends to cause more hangover feelings than whole-extract cannabis oil in my experience. I have had patients who could not tolerate isolated or synthetic THC (such as nabilone and dronabinol) but who then did very well with a full-extract cannabis oil with THC, without side effects. This is the beauty of herbal synergy: the plant chemicals work together to produce a gentler, more balanced effect than you get by pulling out just the THC and putting it into a pill on its own.

What about for sleep apnoea? Some small studies on synthetic THC drugs suggest that THC may have some short-term benefit, but more research is needed to see what the long-term results might be.[28]

Other self-reported data on people using cannabis to help with sleep concluded that cannabis with THC on the whole did seem to improve sleep as well as reduce daytime tiredness.[29, 30] However, as with the other studies above, conclusions were limited due to factors like small sample sizes and huge variations in the type of cannabinoids or cannabis used.

How to use CBD wellness products (hemp CBD) for sleep and rest support

As we have established already, using just CBD without other lifestyle changes and expecting it to knock you out in the same way as a sleeping pill is unlikely to be effective. I have come across people who do use CBD for this purpose and feel they sleep better, but this seems to work best for people whose sleep is mostly affected by anxiety and/or high stress. However, I find it is most beneficial to use CBD alongside other 'sleepy herbs'. These should be taken an hour or so before bedtime, and a CBD oil should be used throughout the day to lower stress and anxiety levels . It is essential to address most sleep problems over the entire 24-hour cycle, and not just immediately before sleep, since brain anxiety and stress levels can impair the normal nervous system wind-down or cause spikes in stress hormone levels, creating what I call brain–sleep barriers.

Starting dose

Try to look for a full-spectrum or broad-spectrum CBD oil rich in myrcene, which tends to be sedating and calming. Because CBD immediately before bedtime on its own may make you feel more alert, the best thing to do is to try using it throughout the day for stress and brain anxiety reduction. Start with 5–10 mg first thing in the morning, repeat the dose at midday/early afternoon (12–2 p.m.) and again at dinner time for a total of 15–30 mg/day. If you are using CBD for anxiety or another indication, see the relevant chapter for more details on titrating up.

Remember: there is no specific perfect dose that works for everyone exactly the same. Each person's endocannabinoid system balance is unique, so self-titration is the name of the game. Take a 'start low, go slow' approach and experiment with taking it at different times in the evening to see what your body likes best. You can track your sleep and how well rested you feel using a sleep app on your phone, or if you are tech-averse, a simple pen and paper sleep journal.

How to use medical cannabis products for sleep

If you have already tried hemp CBD wellness products and not noticed it helping your sleep, try adding in the 'sleepy herbs' and body scanning meditation practice. If you still need help, especially if you also have another symptom or issue where medical cannabis may help, such as pain, neurological symptoms, headaches, anxiety, women's health issues, etc. (see the relevant chapter in this book!), a small dose of THC-containing medical cannabis can be helpful. Only try this under the supervision of a doctor and, of course, if medical cannabis (containing THC) is legal where you live.

- Look for calming terpenes like myrcene and linalool.
- CBN, which is low in raw cannabis but higher in older cannabis

flower and oils as a breakdown product of THC, may enhance the sedative and pain-relieving qualities of the other cannabinoids.[31]

- Start with 2 mg of THC in the form of a cannabis oil an hour before bedtime.
- Slowly increase the dose every few days depending on your response (you can use a simple journal on paper for the low-tech option or a smart watch sleep tracker or app such as WHOOP[32] for additional info). Try to stay below 10 mg of THC if sleep is the primary reason for using it, in order to minimise the risk of disrupting REM sleep (unless this decrease in REM is desired as part of a doctor-led treatment for PTSD).

Vaporising cannabis flowers for trouble falling asleep

- If your main issue is actually getting to sleep, vaporised cannabis flower can be tried instead of an oil, since it works faster and wears off within a few hours. If you have trouble with waking up at night, fragmented sleep or staying asleep, oil or capsules are better because the flower effects will wear off too quickly. If you have tried an oil or capsule and felt hung-over or groggy in the morning, you can try changing from oil to flower before bedtime.
- Start by trying a balanced strain with equal amounts of CBD and THC to start with, to buffer the THC. If you are more experienced with THC already, you can choose a flower product with higher THC and lower CBD (a 1:5 or even 1:10 CBD to THC ratio).
- Choose a product labelled as indica and with dominant terpenes of myrcene and linalool.
- Avoid products labelled as sativas or with activating daytime dominant terpenes such as D-limonene (see Chapter Five for details).
- Start with a very small (matchstick-head-sized amount) for each session. Start with one inhalation.
- See Chapter Five for detailed cannabis vaporising instructions.

CHAPTER TWELVE

MANAGING PAIN

Chronic pain affects up to half of the entire UK population, or an estimated just under 28 million people.[1]

Chronic pain is defined as persistent pain that carries on for longer than three months, and is most commonly associated with conditions such as low back pain and arthritis. However, it can be pain from any source, in any part of the body. It may also start after surgery or an injury, where the acute pain of the initial event just doesn't go away. Some types of chronic pain can start out of the blue without a traumatic injury too, especially stress and strain-related back and neck pain, so common in our sitting-all-day culture.

Chronic pain is a huge quality-of-life problem affecting well over a hundred million people in the US each year, more than cancer, diabetes and heart disease combined. It is the most common cause of disability in America.[2] Although it can affect any age group, the older we get, the more likely we are to suffer from it. The baby boomers are now young seniors, and chronic pain is one of the biggest health issues they face. This generation does not want to become disabled by pain like their parents were, or rely on potent painkillers that cause a whole host of side effects.

My mum, a professional dancer who still teaches at the age of 68, has never taken pain pills despite a little arthritis and occasional back pain. But she is open to trying something natural like CBD (and she has) – why not if there is no downside? Like most of her friends, she wants to change the ageing story, and not being in pain is a huge factor in continuing to be active and healthy into your older years. The cannabis and CBD health revolution is part of the solution to chronic pain and ageing well without the scary side effects of opioids and other prescription pain medications. Around half of my patients are in this over-55 age group or older, and in fact I have one patient of 96 who now uses topical cannabis as the only treatment for his arthritis and other muscle aches and pains. There are multiple published studies demonstrating that cannabis can help with chronic pain and reducing opioid use. In the 2017 US National Academics report, pain is one of the medical problems with the strongest supporting published research evidence for medical cannabis. It is also one of the most common reasons people take CBD wellness products from hemp.

The pain is in the brain too

Chronic pain of all shapes, sizes and varieties is the most common reason why people try CBD and cannabis medicine through self-purchase of CBD wellness products. It is also the most common reason why people are referred to see me for medical cannabis. Without proper management, chronic pain can disrupt livelihoods, hobbies, energy levels and sleep, and strain or even break relationships. It is very hard to be your best self when your brain and body are using most of their bandwidth trying to cope with constant pain. Chronic pain is also interwoven with mental health issues like anxiety and depression. In some cases, it can actually cause these issues, or if they are already there, make them much worse. The issue is that, with most forms of pain that become chronic, the pain is no longer confined to a specific body part. Instead it has become wired in our brains and our nervous systems. Chronic pain creates a constant stress burden that sucks up resources and both mental and physical energy, and the nervous system cannot easily return to a state of rest. I have found that treating chronic pain effectively, even if you can't cure the originating source, is one of the most important and powerful things you can do to drastically improve a person's quality of life.

The traditional Western medical approach to pain is what I like to call the sledgehammer approach. You have the pain drugs like anti-inflammatories, which can help if the pain is more acute and there is inflammation. However, in chronic pain often they may not be effective and they can cause gut side effects. And you have opioids like morphine, which can slightly dampen the pain but whose main function is convincing our brains not to care about it so much. This effect of not minding the pain is good for short-term severe pain, but over time opioids can cause addiction and stop working. They can also create more problems, such as general apathy and low mood, alongside severe constipation and gut issues. The usually well-intended over-prescription of opioids like morphine and fentanyl for chronic low back pain and other chronic pain conditions have contributed to an opioid crisis. But at least it works on the pain, right? Unfortunately not: opioids have been proven to have poor results on chronic pain, not to mention massive side effects and even fatalities. The problem until cannabis came along was that opioids were the only option left for people in severe pain. There's also the surgery approach, often tried for back and knee pain, but unfortunately many of these surgeries do not lead to improved pain long-term, and sometimes can even cause more pain or new types of pain post-operation. While both these approaches have their place, and work well for sources of pain that are acute or can be fixed easily by surgery, most chronic pain conditions are not so simply solved, and the reason for this is that chronic pain is complicated.

There are specific areas of our brain that process pain, as well as areas and brain networks that can become hard-wired to either make pain worse (pain-enhancing brain networks) or reduce it (pain-reducing brain networks). In those experiencing chronic pain, the circuits that enhance pain can get ramped up. In addition to these areas, other parts of the brain get involved in chronic pain too. These are areas that deal with fear, anxiety, mood, learning and emotion. So you can see that the picture gets more complicated than just 'the pain in my knee'. The integrative medicine approach to chronic pain looks at the holistic picture of the pain experience and how we can change the brain pain alongside the chronic pain. Plant cannabinoids are a very useful tool to help do this.

The endocannabinoid system, cannabis and CBD for pain

Cannabis is the single most helpful medicine I have ever used for chronic pain. I have seen it transform the lives of thousands of people as part of an integrative approach. The reason it works so well is that our endocannabinoid system is intimately involved in regulating the brain pain networks, as well as the pain in nerves throughout the body, and even localised body pain in joints and tissues. Adding plant cannabinoids interrupts the pain messages through a multitude of different chemical and brain messenger pathways at both types of cannabinoid receptors (CB1 and CB2).[3] Both THC and CBD as well as other minor cannabinoids and terpenes get in on the pain-busting action.[4] As we know from Chapter Four, cannabinoid receptors are everywhere: the brain, spinal cord[5] and most body tissues, nerve cells, immune cells and major organs all have them.[6] This wide reach helps explain why cannabis works for all the different sorts of chronic pain – something no other pain drug yet invented can do.

It has been shown to work on:

- Neuropathic (nerve) pain – where the pain is in the nerve itself, such as after a direct injury to a nerve or from a process like diabetes (diabetic neuropathy).
- Somatic (body) pain – from a muscle or skeletal system/soft tissue or joint (such as arthritis or muscular pain).
- Psychogenic pain – where there is a brain stress network component in addition to a physical component, such as in tension headaches, where stress, anxiety and fear brain pathways worsen the muscle tension and spasm in a vicious cycle of intensifying headaches.
- Central sensitivity pain – where the brain's pain networks become so sensitive that even non-painful things start to register as pain, such as in complex regional pain syndrome and other chronic pain disorders where the pain is out of proportion to the original injury (ramped-up brain pain, as I like to call it).

Plant cannabinoids can change not only how our brain processes pain, but also our emotional and behavioural brain reactions to it.[7] When our brain areas of emotion and mood become involved in the pain response, this is known as the suffering of the chronic pain experience. It is a very real part of chronic pain, and 'just thinking positively' does not work to counter it. Because cannabis works on both these elements of pain, unlike the other pain medications we use in Western medicine, it is a very powerful tool.

Exercise also activates the analgesic (pain relief) effects of the endocannabinoid system,[8] which is one of the reasons why staying active is so important if you have chronic pain. However, for most of my patients, before they start cannabis, they are in too much pain or too deconditioned (out of shape) to want to or be able to exercise properly. This situation leads to a vicious cycle of no exercise leading to more weight gain and weakness, which brings more pain, making it harder to exercise, and in turn contributing to low energy and mood. Cannabis helps them break this cycle.

Mary's story: breaking the pain, fatigue and weight-gain cycle

Mary was 60 years old, and until 15 years ago when her back trouble started, she had always been fairly fit and healthy. She was now almost housebound due to inoperable severe back pain, which limited her ability to walk and even sit for any period of time in the car. She had accumulated more than 10 medications related to her pain condition when I saw her for the first visit. These included opioids, muscle relaxants, various nerve pain medications, benzodiazepines, sleeping pills and other drugs for the side effects of these pills. She was depressed, in pain and very overweight. She had gained 80 pounds over the course of 15 years of severe pain and her only comfort was food. She used to be very active and walk in the woods near her home every day with her dog. Now she was in too much pain and too groggy from the opioids and other medications to do that any longer.

She had never smoked cannabis or used it recreationally, but a friend had tried a high-CBD oil for pain and convinced her to try it, which she did. To her surprise, she found it helped her pain and didn't make her feel stoned, so she thought maybe she should investigate it further with a doctor. She was worried what the neighbours would think, however, and was concerned when we first met that she might need to smoke or inhale it, which was just not something she was comfortable with.

We started her on cannabis first in oil form and then capsules, which was totally discreet. Over a 12-month period she lost 65 pounds, started walking again (with her new puppy!), got off her opioid painkillers, her benzodiazepines and her high-dose anti-inflammatory drugs as well as her sleeping pills. She said that she felt like she had her life back again, something she had never imagined possible. She was so grateful she had found medical cannabis, but she also felt angry that no doctor had offered it to her sooner – why did they let her suffer for 10 years when this was available as a treatment option?

Mary's story is one of thousands I have heard from the patients I have seen and treated with cannabis for chronic pain. It's not uncommon for people not just to feel better and have less pain, but also to lose significant amounts of weight, improve blood sugar control (in diabetes and pre-diabetes) and return to work again after years of being on disability for pain. In those experiencing serious depression along with their pain condition, this can also go into remission, allowing them to experience life once again with joy. Cannabis is the catalyst that makes these things possible by helping with pain, mood and sleep. Furthermore, under medical supervision, it helps people to wean down and even in some cases off opioids and other medications completely that were offering minimal benefit at significant cost in terms of side effects.

At least half of my patients, like Mary, have never smoked or tried cannabis in any shape or form before coming to see me for medical cannabis. They take this step feeling they've reached the end of the line after trying every pain relief drug and non-drug approach on the planet, with limited success. Many want to get off their opioid painkillers and other pills that they are currently reliant on because they are tired of the horrible side effects. They also get less pain relief the longer they take them. Doctors often prescribe two or three more medications just to cope with the side effects of the first one. It is not a nice situation and they feel fed up.

The local herbalist cannabis guy

In both the UK and Canada, long before medical cannabis was available by prescription, people were self-medicating for pain through what I call 'knowing a guy'. In the best-case scenario, if you were not a smoker of cannabis, you would find through word of mouth a cannabis guy who would be able to provide some sort of homemade tincture to take by mouth. Where I worked as a doctor in rural British Columbia, most communities had a least one cannabis oil/tincture guy like this. While practising in one such community, I met a self-taught herbalist who grew cannabis of various strains and made tinctures for medicinal uses. Most of the local people knew of him, and he had helped some of my patients with chronic pain, using his tinctures as an alternative to morphine and opioid painkillers.

I had one elderly patient with very advanced cancer and terrible bone pain who confided to me that he was using a cannabis tincture. He found that with it, he was able to take less of his very strong painkillers, which left him feeling groggy, dizzy and generally out of it. Although I couldn't prescribe the tincture for him, as it wasn't an approved medical cannabis product (and we didn't actually know how much THC and CBD was in it), I found he had great relief in his final days. He used it successfully to ease his suffering, maximise his quality of life and be more present with his friends and family.

This was one of my earlier experiences with cannabis in a medical context, and it started to pique my interest in cannabis as a botanical medicine worthy of consideration alongside, and complementing, Western medicine. This East-meets-West approach was especially useful for pain, anxiety, insomnia, chronic fatigue and other symptoms and conditions where Western medicine pills had often been tried and failed, or had worked partially but still had room for improvement. It also applied when patients desired a natural option that would still likely be effective without significant side effects.

I become a pain patient of cannabis

While I was in Bali setting up our brain wellness centre, I got hit by a motorcycle, flew through the air and badly injured my left wrist and hand. With no other injuries or head knocks, I was extremely lucky. However, in addition to fracturing my scaphoid bone, I had completely blown the ligament that essentially holds two of the hand bones together so the wrist joint works properly.

After two painful, and not wholly successful, operations, I was left with nerve damage and early arthritis due to the bones rubbing together where the ligament used to be. I saw three top surgeons on three different continents and all gave me pretty abysmal news. They said that if I rode my beloved road bike or did any sort of yoga pose with weight in the hands (such as a downward dog or chaturanga), I would likely have debilitating arthritis and pain that would get worse over time, to the point where I would eventually have to have my hand fused to my wrist and have a permanently disabled left hand.

I was offered multiple pain medications and advised that I would likely need them for life. I decided that this option was not for me; I was not willing to accept that prognosis or treatment. Instead, I would use every ounce of my mind-body medicine training and herbal medicine background to find some other way to cope and regain as much function in my hand as possible.

I had to figure something out quickly, though, because the burning nerve pain was waking me up multiple times each night. During the day, the constant low-grade ache would sometimes become acutely painful, which made working with my hands, even just typing my patient chart notes, very difficult.

I did neuro-mirroring exercises, visualisation and biofeedback, but the final piece was finding cannabis medicine.

I was attending the annual American Academy of Integrative Medicine (AIHM) conference in San Diego, which attracts the top mainstream medical doctors with an interest in integrative medicine from all over the world. (It is my favourite medical conference by far, and I had the privilege of speaking there on the topic of cannabis medicine a few years later.) One of my colleagues, Dr Scott Shannon, a top integrative psychiatrist in the US and a mentor in all things holistic mental health, started chatting with me in one of the breaks. I mentioned my hand injury, which was in a fancy-looking custom-made comfort splint. He suggested I check out one of the conference vendors, a legal medical cannabis company, and get a sample of one of their topical high-CBD balms for my nerve pain.

I was quite sceptical (and a bit worried about the idea of cannabis at a respectable medical conference!), but I did seek them out and they very kindly gave me a free container of cannabis topical for pain, instructing me to rub it in three to four times a day, or more if I could manage it.

I was in San Diego for seven days and I started the balm on day one, keeping it with me throughout the day at the conference and dutifully applying it every few hours. By day three, the nerve pain was no longer waking me up – it felt like a miracle! By day seven, it just didn't hurt any more, at least not enough to notice it. I realised I had not thought about my hand all day for the first time in months.

This experience was my tipping point with medical cannabis. When I returned to Canada, I realised that was it, I had to get with the programme and start using cannabis to help my patients who were being failed by other drug therapies. If I approached cannabis the same way I did every other thing else in medicine, using a scientific method and matching the product, strain and plant to the patient as much as possible, I knew there was much that could be done with this plant medicine.

Kim's story

Kim was a professional guitarist who had been a part of a successful professional touring group until she developed an aggressive form of arthritis that attacked her hands. This made playing the guitar nearly impossible by the time she reached her 40th birthday. She fell into a deep depression, feeling she had lost her livelihood, her passion and her means of expression all in one go.

When I saw her, she was severely depressed and rarely left the house, feeling that her life lacked any real joy. She was on painkillers, anti-inflammatories, sleeping pills, anxiety pills and antidepressants, yet despite this cocktail of drugs, her quality of life hadn't improved.

We started working together and I put Kim on high-CBD, low-THC cannabis, using oils under the tongue, one for day and one for night, as well as cannabis flower with both THC and CBD inhaled with a vaporiser for her severe fatigue and acute pain spasms. Every month she got a bit better: she looked me in the eye, she smiled, and at the six-month visit, I found that she was engaged, joking and relaxed.

Kim told me this was how she used to be before she got sick. She said her entire life was changing: not just her inflammation, pain, mood and sleep (which were all dramatically better), but her hope for the future and her happiness. She started to get her mojo back for the first time in ten years. One day, she showed up on my patient schedule even though she wasn't due to see me for another two months. I thought something had gone wrong and that she'd had a setback, but when I logged on to the video call, she had arranged a surprise for me. She unveiled her newly renovated recording studio and played a mini concert for me for a few minutes, smiling ear to ear.

She was playing again for the first time in five years and got her first professional gig after almost seven years of not working. I was moved to tears. In many years of practising medicine, both conventional and holistic, I had never had anything like that happen.

Jack's story

Jack was a patient of mine with multiple medical issues and a type of severe pain disorder called complex regional pain syndrome, which left him with near-constant throbbing, burning pain in his leg. When I first saw him, he was on ten different medications to manage the pain (and secondary anxiety from being in pain 24/7!), all with quite bad side effects. However, he did not want to take a lot of THC during the day because he was worried about it impairing his driving or making him feel intoxicated. So we added a high-CBD, low-THC cannabis oil as his daytime base, and over a period of months, this improved things and he slowly was able to come off many of his other pain and anxiety pills.

However, on top of the constant throbbing, burning pain, he also had debilitating acute spasm and pain attacks or episodes that would come on without any warning, and pills or cannabis oils didn't work fast enough. It was these acute attacks where vaporised cannabis helped the most, and gave him almost immediate relief, stopping an attack in 5–10 minutes rather than it lasting hours and confining him to bed for half a day. He liked this option too because although he could vaporise a higher amount of THC to stop the pain quickly, it wore off faster so he did not feel impaired to drive a few hours later. This proved an effective, convenient and flexible way for him to take a more potent cannabis medicine on the days where he needed it, without having to use a high-THC oil, which can last for up to six hours.

How to use CBD wellness products (hemp CBD) for chronic pain

Many people who have severe chronic pain may have already tried hemp CBD oil on their own and not noticed much of a change. In my experience, most people in this category, regardless of the source of pain, may need some THC. Even a small dose using a high-CBD medical cannabis product (i.e. with 1% THC) is sometimes enough for pain relief, especially if there is an inflammatory component to the pain. That being said, I have also become aware of many cases where people have used an over-the-counter high-quality, hemp-based CBD product for a variety of chronic pain conditions and it has worked for them for both pain and inflammation without needing to graduate to any prescription products with THC, even in some cases allowing them to stop other prescription pain pills. CBD on its own has been found to have a profound anti-inflammatory effect, and reduces nerve pain in animal models, which is likely similar in humans, although we lack these specific studies as of yet.[9, 10]

- Use a full-spectrum or broad-spectrum CBD oil.
- Look for anti-inflammatory terpenes:
    - beta-caryophyllene – also in black pepper; has a woody/spicy aroma

- myrcene – smells like hops/earthy/peppery, and is sedating so good for night-time pain (may be too sedating for daytime); also has anti-inflammatory activity.

Starting dose and titrating up

Starting doses for pain can vary from person to person, but in general, try starting with 10 mg of CBD first thing in the morning, again at midday/early afternoon (12–2 p.m.) and a third dose at dinner time for a total of 30 mg/day. Stay at this dose for a few days to a week or so or slowly increase the dose every few days depending on your pain response and preference.

- Is the pain level improving?
- Are other symptoms improving (inflammation, stiffness, achiness, anxiety, fatigue, mood)?
- Is it still bad at a certain time of day (e.g. worse when you wake up or in the evening)?
- Are you still having trouble getting to sleep or staying asleep due to the pain waking you?

Score your pain level each day in the morning, afternoon and evening (after dinner) on a scale from 0–10, where 0 = pain free, 10 = unbearable/worst pain imaginable, and write down the results in a symptom tracker, which can be a simple diary.

You can slowly keep increasing the dose each week until symptoms improve. If you do not notice any change in the first few weeks, do not give up, as CBD's effects on the nervous system and brain pain are often gradual over the weeks and months after you start taking it. I do find it works best when you take it consistently over a long period rather than only when you are having a pain crisis. For most people it does not have an immediate effect like a painkiller drug; normally the results are more subtle and it is best used to decrease chronic pain over time.

If you reach 60 mg total per day of CBD, stay here for another 4–6 weeks before increasing the dose again. For inflammatory pain, higher doses may be needed, especially if you are not adding any

THC from a prescription cannabis product. For pain, long acting slow release forms of CBD that are more absorbable, such as transdermal patches, are a great option in such cases where CBD oil is not sufficient, although not yet widely available.

Remember: there is no specific perfect dose that works for everyone exactly the same. Each person's endocannabinoid system balance is unique, so self-titration is the name of the game.

For maintenance: non-cannabis helpers to add

The lowest effective CBD dose is recommended to reduce the cost and number of bottles of CBD oil needed per month. Once you reach a dose that is helping you, then you can start adding in other anti-pain and inflammation busters to help get even better effects and start to really rewire the brain's chronic pain pathways in the longer term:

- mindfulness meditation
- anti-inflammatory herbs: turmeric, curcumin, boswellia and bromelain
- non-weight-bearing exercise for joint pain, such as elliptical trainer, swimming and power-walking, as well as meditative movement such as gentle yoga and t'ai chi

How to use medical cannabis products for chronic pain

If you have already tried hemp CBD and not noticed a huge change, adding some THC can be hugely beneficial for more difficult pain issues. The CBD can buffer the psychoactivity and possible side effects of THC and also works in synergy with it on pain through both endocannabinoid system receptor pathways and other chemical pathways, like the serotonin system and other non-endocannabinoid pain networks.[11, 12] Only try this under the supervision of a doctor and, of course, if medical cannabis (containing THC) is legal where you live.

- For daytime pain: start with a high-CBD cannabis oil as your base. Choose a product high in CBD and very low in THC (e.g. CBD to THC ratio of 20:1). Look for anti-inflammatory terpenes such as beta-caryophyllene for anti-inflammatory action and other good daytime terpenes (see Chapter Five for details).
- Average starting dose: 5–10 mg 3x/day with meals: so with breakfast, lunch and dinner.
- For night-time pain and sleep disruption: it is very common for chronic pain to disturb sleep and proper rest and to get worse in the evening, possibly due to changes in cytokine levels. Many patients are at first unaware of how badly they sleep, and it's only when they're sleeping better that they notice how fatigued and unrested they felt in the morning previously. That is why I always treat night pain and sleep from the get-go with a night-time cannabis medicine dose using higher THC, unless there is a contraindication (see Chapter Six for details).
  - Start with a balanced (i.e. 1:1 ratio) or a high-THC, low-CBD strain cannabis oil.
  - Look for calming terpenes like myrcene and linalool.
  - CBN, which is low in raw cannabis but higher in older cannabis flower and oils as a breakdown product of THC,[13] may enhance the sedative and pain-relieving qualities of the other cannabinoids.[14]
  - Start with 2 mg of THC and take an hour before bedtime.
- These dose ranges start at less than the dose for the hemp CBD wellness products because all medical cannabis oils (even the high-CBD oils) have some THC above the hemp level of 0.2/0.3%. This often makes it work better at lower doses.
- For both day and night, stay at this dose for 1–2 weeks or slowly increase the dose every few days depending on your pain response and preference.
- If your pain is worse at a certain time of day, increase the previous dose; for example, if your pain gets worse around 4–5 p.m., try increasing your lunchtime dose to get ahead of the pain later in the day.

- Because there are varying amounts of THC in these oils depending on the exact one you are using, slowly titrate the dose up by a few mg each week as needed to get relief, tracking your symptoms and your response as before.

How to use vaporising cannabis flowers for pain

This is the best mode of delivery for stopping acute pain in the moment, or muscle spasms or headache attacks that come on suddenly. It should be an add-on to a base of cannabis oil generally, not the primary mode of use, in order to minimise side effects and avoid a roller coaster of THC levels.

- Start with high-CBD, low-THC flowers especially if you are new to THC, because THC from vaporised cannabis hits the brain faster than oils by mouth.
- If this has no effect, you can try a balanced strain, with equal amounts of CBD to THC (i.e. 1:1).
- Start with a matchstick-head-sized amount, especially if it is a strain with more THC.
- See Chapter Five for detailed cannabis vaporising instructions.

Topicals: when and how to use

Topicals can be helpful for localised areas of pain, especially joint pain in small close-to-the-surface joints like knees, wrists and hands as well as ankles and foot/toe arthritis. Muscle balms with CBD and menthol may also be helpful for aches and pains and are extremely safe. They can be applied to painful areas of muscle any time, but may work best after a hot shower when pores are open, and when using a topical that contains menthol and linalool to help the CBD penetrate slightly better into the skin. CBD has more penetrability than THC when used topically, but topical THC may also help inflammation (where legally available) and pain. Hemp CBD-based topicals may help with arthritis pain too, to variable degrees, and although studies are lacking, many people report anecdotally that it has helped with muscular aches and pains as well.

> **NOTE**
>
> Topicals are not the same as transdermal patches. For example, a topical CBD product or cream only absorbs into the local skin area vs a transdermal patch is a high-tech way of getting the CBD (and/or THC in the case of medical cannabis) through all the skin layers and into the bloodstream. This is an important distinction.

Multiple animal studies have found that topical CBD preparations have reduced joint swelling. Lower back pain that has a nerve component sometimes also responds at least partly to topicals with CBD, although results vary from person to person and from product to product. For widespread pain, oral or vaporised routes (systemic) are better, but an isolated joint pain may respond well to just topicals or a combination of low-dose oral oils plus topicals. I still regularly use CBD topicals made from hemp on my hand scar and over the joint where I had my injury, and find they give me good relief from occasional pain flares on their own without needing anything else added to them.

Migraines

When it comes to treating migraine headaches and other forms of chronic headache, cannabis can work wonders, but sometimes it takes patience and time to find the right CBD to THC ratio and strain. If the migraines are happening more than twice a month, or they are lasting for an entire day or more, my approach is to start taking a daily oil for prevention or reduction; this is what doctors call a prophylactic treatment.

I start patients with a very low dose (5 mg 2x/day) of a high-CBD, low-THC oil (especially if they are unused to cannabis); or in cases where CBD has already been tried, a very small dose (1–2 mg 2–3x/ day) of a balanced (1:1 ratio) oil. CBD on its own, especially if dosed too high too fast, may actually trigger a migraine in some people, while for others, using a hemp CBD oil daily has reduced their headaches, so again each case is a bit different. I have found this treatment helps, over time, to decrease the frequency and severity of headaches for many people.

For aborting or stopping a migraine, I will add inhaled vaporised cannabis for rescue when a headache has just started or when someone has an aura, right before the pain starts. This is often very useful in patients who are already on high doses of triptans and/or opioid painkillers for rescue migraine pain. Although part of their headache may be a rebound headache from overuse of these drugs, you cannot stop these meds altogether without giving patients an alternative pain solution, otherwise the migraine can become so severe it requires a hospital trip for intravenous drugs to get it under control. This is where using vaporised cannabis comes in handy. As soon as you feel the headache coming on, you vaporise a small amount of cannabis, usually containing both CBD and THC and high in terpenes like beta-caryophyllene and myrcene. It aborts the headache without having to take the other painkillers that may have been causing part of the vicious headache cycle. It is important to note that after using this vaporised cannabis, even though the strains used contain THC, most of my patients say they feel less impaired than by using their previous prescription pain and migraine drugs.

Casey's story: the headache that was ruining her life

Casey was referred to me for her severe headaches. She had been on a waiting list for two years to see a neurologist headache specialist and last year was finally put on the best headache drug cocktail they could offer her. However, despite maximal medical therapy, as it's called, she continued to have debilitating headaches multiple days each week. A busy mum with three kids, her headaches were massively interfering with her life and her feelings about herself as a mum. She had to miss school meetings, concerts and sporting events because of sudden migraine onset which would send her back to bed on short notice. She had also had decided recently to give up her job because she was missing so many days at work due to the headaches, despite loving her role as a creative director in a marketing ad agency. She felt incredibly guilty and even depressed because of the current situation and her inability to get control over it, even doing everything the doctor told her to do. It was a feeling of utter helplessness.

I started working with Casey using a high-CBD, low-THC oil titrated up very slowly over a period of a few months. We also used specific vaporised cannabis strains higher in THC and containing beta-caryophyllene to stop the headache in its tracks before things got really ramped up. After six months, after some playing around with strains and doses, we found the sweet spot. Casey was only getting around one headache a month, lasting for an hour, when her previous headaches had lasted an entire day. She had not missed a single event for her kids in the past two months, which was completely shifting the way she saw herself and her relationship with them. She was also considering going back to work part-time. She told me she felt she was starting to have a life again thanks to medical cannabis.

Cancer pain and chemotherapy-induced neuropathy/pain

We are still at the beginning of our understanding of how different types of cancers in humans respond to different types of cannabis. While animal studies are plentiful, animal models do not always match up to human experience. Because of the different ways each of us is affected by cannabis and the different cannabinoid strains available, I always recommend using the lowest effective dose and consulting with your primary care and oncology team about possible risks and benefits of adding cannabis for pain and side-effect management. They can also advise how it may interact (at least in theory) with the cancer treatment (also see Chapter Six for drug interactions).

While there have been very promising case reports of patients curing themselves of certain cancers using home-made cannabis oils in very high doses when conventional chemotherapy has failed, we need more studies to accurately predict how an individual cancer may respond to cannabinoids, and the doses that are best. Each type of tumour has different receptors and may respond differently. Most preliminary studies, are pointing to low-dose cannabinoids being fairly safe for side-effect management in many types of cancers. In general, I advise against using dried flower (vaporised or smoked cannabis – anything inhaled) in cancer patients who are immuno-compromised (undergoing chemo or radiotherapy or other active treatment) due to the possibility of moulds and biotoxins or bacteria in the flowers. If inhaled routes are preferred, you may try gamma-ir-radiated flower products under a physician's advice, but oral oils or sublingual tinctures are usually best if tolerated. Rectal routes do not seem to lead to as much systemic absorption of THC, but the evidence is very early and scarce and mostly anecdotal, and some people do report this method to be effective. It may offer some relief if a patient cannot tolerate something by mouth or sublingually due to mouth sores.

With cancer pain from the disease itself, such as in advanced cancers where bone pain is an issue, a strain with substantial THC may be most effective, so to buffer against THC side effects I usually start with a 1:1 balanced strain. I prescribe this in an oil form if the pain is constant, or as vaporised cannabis if it is only occasional and comes on without warning and then goes away again.

Studies in animals show that CBD may be protective against chemotherapy-induced nerve pain, and may also help decrease this symptom if it is already occurring.[15]

Neuropathic pain (nerve pain)

For nerve pain of many causes, including diabetic neuropathy, a high-CBD, low-THC variety may work best, based on the CBD-dominant effects on nerve pain (see pp.212–16 above for details on how to take).

Fibromyalgia

As an integrative medicine doctor, I see many patients with fibromy-algia when other doctors (and often naturopaths too) do not know what else to offer them. This is a complex disorder that is not yet fully understood, but we know that it involves the brain, nervous system and likely the immune system too. The pain of fibromyalgia is all too real, despite what many of my unfortunate patients have been told by various doctors before finally getting to me. Frequently they are told that it's all in their head and they just need to see a psychiatrist, or that they are exaggerating. This dismissal of very real and distressing symptoms does not help these patients one little bit, and often just my being able to tell them that this is a real diagnosis brings some relief. After that, of course, it's what we can actually do about it, which is where cannabis and CBD come in.

A number of my patients with fibromyalgia are extremely sensitive to many drugs as well as natural supplements and herbals. Because of this, I start with a micro dose (5 mg 2x/day with a meal), even if using a hemp-based CBD oil with less than 0.2% THC, and slowly increase the dose every few days until an effect on pain and/or fatigue/stiff-ness is noticed. I find that fibromyalgia symptoms respond extremely well to cannabis. Each person is a bit different regarding the ratio of CBD to THC that works best for them, so tracking symptoms and changing the product if no effect is seen after 6–8 weeks is a good way to investigate and discover what works best for you.

Fibromyalgia is thought to be related to migraine headaches and irritable bowel syndrome, and Dr Ethan Russo, an American medical doctor and cannabis researcher, is investigating the concept that they are all linked to an endocannabinoid deficiency. This may explain why adding plant cannabinoids helps people with these illnesses feel nor-mal again even when every other drug or supplement may have failed. Other forms of treatment-resistant central-sensitivity pain syndromes may also respond very well to cannabis for the same reason – see for example Jack's story (pp.211–12 above).

Arthritis/joint pain

As mentioned in the topicals section, small-joint arthritis and local-ised joint pain respond very well to topicals. High-CBD oil by mouth may also be helpful for inflammation and vaporised cannabis for acute pain flare-ups, especially for small joints near the surface of the body such as the knee, ankle, hand and wrist. See Chapter Sixteen for additional information on autoimmune arthritis.

Muscle pain

CBD and cannabis topicals in a muscle rub applied after a hot shower may help ease muscle aches and pains. Many people report improve-ments in muscular aches and pains and quicker recovery after hard workouts when they take high-CBD cannabis oil or even hemp CBD oil. There are not yet any published human studies on this, but in the-ory it makes sense that topicals may be helpful for muscular recovery due to CBD's anti-inflammatory and antioxidant activity. Many pro-fessional athletes are starting to use zero-THC hemp-based CBD oil by mouth and topically to reduce soreness. This reduces the need for the high-dose NSAID anti-inflammatory and opioid drugs often taken after a game in sports like rugby and American football, where contact injuries happen in nearly every game.

Chronic pelvic pain

There have been many anecdotal reports of people using rectal and vaginal cannabis suppositories containing just CBD or a combina-tion of CBD and THC for chronic pelvic pain and related conditions. Despite the fact that based on preliminary research, THC systemic absorption by rectal methods seems to be minimal, I have had patients use high-THC suppositories get a bit of a buzz from the THC that lasted quite a long time – nearly a whole day in some cases. It's unclear if these were just a few very sensitive individuals or if this is an average response to rectal THC, since in theory it is not well absorbed into the bloodstream rectally. It may also be dose-dependent. It is also possible (quite likely) that these products may have localised anti-inflammatory and pain-relieving effects.

In my medical practice, I had a few cases of chronic non-bacterial prostatitis (a painful chronic inflammation of the prostate gland in men, without a known cause), where cannabis suppositories reduced symptoms despite all other interventions and pain medications failing to make much difference. I have had similar reports from friends and emails from women who use vaginal suppositories for menstrual pain (more on this in Chapter Thirteen), even if we lack clinical data as of yet.

CHAPTER THIRTEEN

OPTIMISING WOMEN'S HEALTH

Cannabis has been used as a medicine in women's health for thousands of years, for symptoms ranging from pain in childbirth to period pain. Often it has been administered via inhaled or ingested (as a tincture) methods, but also in some instances via rectal or vaginal routes.[1] However, most accounts about the specifics have been lost in the mists of time and many lack modern research studies, in large part due to the fact that plant medicine is harder to study than drugs and has less of a financial return. The patriarchal history of Western medicine, and a corresponding lack of female physicians, has meant that historically women's health issues were less studied than problems that affected both men and women, or only men. For many years Western medicine gave little consideration to such female-specific conditions as pelvic floor dysfunction, women's cancers and menstrual problems. In 1950 in the UK, only 6% of physicians were women, and things were slow to change for the next decade after that.[2] Thankfully I feel we are now moving towards a more balanced medical landscape for women.

In my medical training, many women's health issues, ranging from hormonal acne to nightmare periods and premenstrual syndrome, were treated first and foremost by suppressing the menstrual cycle and our natural monthly hormonal ebbs and flows with the Pill, instead of looking deeper for underlying causes or providing an explanation for why these symptoms might be happening. I am a proponent of empowering and supporting women with whatever choice they feel is best for them (some people love the Pill and find it works for them). I also believe they should be informed about all of their options, including natural ones. Teaching all women about our menstrual cycle and how our hormones work is of extreme importance in helping us understand our own bodies. Also important is understanding how factors like stress, sleep, food and our emotional health can affect our hormones. When our bodies and hormonal cycles are no longer a mystery, it can stop that feeling of being at war with ourselves and at the mercy of our bodies. First it's our menstrual cycle and then later perimenopause, menopause and beyond as our bodies and hormone cycles change. I have had countless female patients over the years who told me I was the first doctor they had ever seen who explained the issues they had been facing in detail rather than insisting they needed to just go on the Pill. I have also found that many women decide to stop the Pill after decades and then struggle to understand their natural cycle again, since it has been suppressed for most of their adult life.

It's not surprising that cannabis seems to help with many women's health-related symptoms, as there are cannabinoid receptors throughout the female reproductive tract, from our uterus (where they are most concentrated) to our vagina and vulva. The star player of the endocannabinoid system is called AEA and is produced in the ovaries. It plays a role in every phase of our menstrual cycle:[3] in the follicular phase (folliculogenesis and follicle maturation) and in ovulation (release of an egg), as well as in pregnancy. It appears that THC has a very similar effect on the body to our naturally produced AEA, although we are still discovering exactly what plant THC (and CBD) does at different phases of the menstrual cycle.

It's notable that we currently do not have much in the way of human studies of THC on the hormonal cycles of women, yet we have dozens of studies on the effects of THC on sexual function in men! We do, however, know that there are cannabinoid receptors in the parts of the brain that control the ovarian hormones (the hypothalamus),[4] as well as in the anterior pituitary, so even from a brain level, the ECS is pulling the strings when it comes to our hormone cycles.

One study done in female cows showed that the endocannabinoid receptors and enzyme levels were different in the first half (follicular phase before ovulation, e.g. days 1–14) to the second half (the luteal phase, after ovulation but before the first day of the period) of the menstrual cycle. So our endocannabinoids follow the same pattern as other hormones like oestrogen and progesterone, in that the levels change depending on what phase of our cycle we are in.

What we have seen so far from women using cannabis for issues ranging from period problems to enhancing sexual enjoyment (see Chapter Fourteen) is that these cannabinoid receptors are involved in how we experience both pleasure as well as pain and discomfort from our reproductive organs. The endocannabinoid system may even be a greater influence than our sex hormones on food cravings before our periods (something I like to deal with by having a stash of dark chocolate in a lockbox to prevent my husband eating it all first!).[5]

What also seems clear in the research to date is that, just like with disorders of other major body systems, dysregulation of the endo-cannabinoid system is associated with a variety of women's health issues ranging from period problems and PMS to reproductive cancers and fertility, and we still have a lot to learn about the details.[6]

Period problems: painful periods, cramping, bloating and PMS

When it comes to dealing with period pain, I've heard about everything from CBD on tampons to using topical 'tummy' creams and vaginal CBD and cannabis suppositories. These potential uses of CBD and cannabis currently lack controlled trials and published research studies, yet many women anecdotally report benefits. Many conventional gynaecologists dismiss this as a placebo effect, but I find that highly unlikely to be the case considering the long history of cannabis in traditional use, as well as the proven cannabinoid recep-tors throughout the reproductive tract. Unfortunately in Western medicine when doctors don't understand something they are quick to dismiss it, rather than admit they don't know or that it could be possible. It drives me crazy, because if I've learned anything from over ten years of practising medicine, it's that the more I learn, the more I realise we don't know yet! We do know, however, that THC is a muscle relaxant and both THC and CBD are potent anti-inflammatories, which could explain how they may improve symptoms like cramps, bloating and other period-related symptoms that may have an inflammatory and muscle spasm component.

When I was at university, one of my friend's housemates was a traditional herbalist and used to grow a few cannabis plants in their back garden (the bong alarm clock house!). She would harvest these, hang them to dry in the rafters of her attic bedroom and then make topical balms for her clients with menstrual pain and period problems. She had many satisfied customers, who all found her through local word of mouth. In my medical practice, many patients told me of going to a dispensary to get a topical balm for rubbing onto the abdomen, and claimed it helped them with their period pain and cramps. It did not put them in danger of intoxication from inhaled or ingested THC (this was before the hemp CBD wellness movement, so they didn't yet have the option of CBD oil), and is likely a very safe way to try both CBD and topical cannabis products for period issues, with little risk of altering your female hormone levels.

In more recent years, CBD hemp oils, CBD-infused tampons and vaginal suppositories – both hemp CBD (legal over the counter in the UK) and THC-containing versions (in some US states and in Canada without a prescription) – are becoming more popular. At the time of writing there are no published studies on these types of products in any peer-reviewed academic research journals (and believe me, I looked). It is therefore impossible to say what is definitely happening with these products used inside the vagina. All we can say is that given the long history of use of cannabis in many forms for women's health, and even in pregnancy, it appears to have low toxicity, but the exact extent of the effects of these products in terms of affecting hormone cycles and fertility factors (like ovulation) are unknown. Again, doctors hate saying we don't know, often preferring to claim something is bad if unsure just to cover our butts, but the truth is we don't know all the answers yet when it comes to CBD and cannabis tampons and women's health products for vaginal use.

One of the issues is that the main source of information about these products comes from the companies that are making them, based on customer feedback, rather than published, peer-reviewed research. That doesn't mean the products don't work or that the companies are lying about people claiming they do. However, it does mean that we still don't know exactly how they affect us yet and what the actual risks are (although they're likely pretty low). This is also one of the things I find interesting about the way cannabis medicine and cannabis for wellness has evolved in the recent modern era. The movement has come from consumers, patients and self-use experimentation, more grassroots- and often female-led, as opposed to the top-down way drugs are tested. This has its challenges when it comes to providing evidence doctors will accept, but at the same time, it has led to a decrease in stigma around the cannabis plant and its medicinal value. The studies looking so far at the effects of cannabis on women's hormones have been limited to inhaled or ingested products, not vaginal routes, so again there are more questions than answers for the new wave of products. I hope the results many women are reporting will lead to research and more definitive answers in the near future.

Period problems, as well as most other women's health and hormone issues, are made worse by chronic unchecked stress, which cannabinoids and CBD-rich products in particular can help with, as they can help regulate the stress response (see Chapter Eight for details).

In addition to cannabis and CBD, if you suffer from any kind of PMS or painful periods, I also recommend following what is known as a hormone-balancing diet. This is a diet that is high in both soluble and insoluble fibre, low in refined carbohydrates, high in healthy fats and low-glycaemic-index foods and plant-rich. When I work with my patients and clients one to one, I often add botanicals such as ashwagandha and chasteberry as well as magnesium, vitamin D and B vitamins, as these nutritional factors all stacked up can make a big difference when you stick to them over many months.

Period pain

Over 90% of menstruating women suffer to some degree with period pain (or dysmenorrhoea, as we doctors know it), and it can range from mildly annoying to full-blown, day-cancelling, stuck-in-bed pain. One of the contributing factors seems to be higher levels of certain types of chemicals called prostaglandins. These chemicals are elevated in women who get bad period pain,[7] causing constriction of blood vessels and contractions of the uterus as well as inflammation, and can hypersensitise nerves in the pelvic region to pain. CBD and THC can inhibit these chemicals,[8] and so it makes sense that both CBD wellness products and medical cannabis can help with period pain, often more effectively than any other pill or non-drug-based approach.

In my medical practice, I have successfully prescribed medical cannabis (mainly via oils or vaporised) for severe period pain for patients who had limited success with other drugs, such as prescription anti-inflammatories and opioid painkillers. Those heavy-duty pharmaceuticals also come with strong side effects, and patients report being glad to stop taking them.

Using CBD for period pain

CBD is a potent anti-inflammatory. The best conventional drug treatment for period pain is strong NSAIDs, or anti-inflammatory drugs (probably due to the effect on prostaglandins and other inflammatory pathways). To get a similar benefit from CBD without the side effects of the drugs, you can try taking a good-quality CBD oil and look for one containing beta-caryophyllene (an anti-inflammatory), starting 7–10 days before your period (if you also get PMS symptoms) and experimenting to find your optimal dose over a few cycles or so. Or you can start just 2 days before your period if your main issue is cramps and period pain just on your bleeding days. You have to experiment to see what works best for your body, since there are no published reports to go on. You could start with 10–20 mg of CBD three times a day. Some people report benefit from higher doses (80–100 mg/day total dose), but start with 30 mg/day to keep costs down, and see where your sweet spot is. As always, start low, go slow.

Using medical cannabis for period pain

If you have this option available legally where you are under doctor supervision, and the CBD-only option has been tried for three full menstrual cycles at a high dose without success, there are two options for additional relief adding products with THC:

1. For chronic period pain that lasts several days, start dosing 2 days before the start of your period. One hour before bedtime, try taking a very small dose of a cannabis oil containing both THC and CBD in an even ratio, starting with around 4 mg (giving you 2 mg of CBD and 2 mg of THC). If you still have pain in the morning, try taking another 4 mg dose (if you are new to THC, try it first on a weekend or day at home in case of impairment). Increase the dose each day by 1–2 mg as needed until the pain is over (usually by the end of your period). If the balanced oil makes you feel more awake, you can try just using a high THC low CBD oil in a 2 mg dose to start before bedtime. In the future for this type of chronic pain around your period that seems to be constant for a few days, a transdermal medical cannabis or CBD patch which is slow release into the bloodstream over a few days may also be a good option, once more widely available.

2. If your cramps are only mild and come on suddenly but don't last all day (i.e. you just need occasional rescue pain relief), you can try an inhaled cannabis product, again with a balanced THC to CBD ratio. Start with one inhalation (see Chapter Five for how to dose inhaled cannabis and Chapter Twelve for the best strains for acute pain flares). This method of medicating is also useful if you have menstrual migraine headaches (see Chapter Twelve).

Using topicals for period pain

Both CBD balms from hemp and topicals containing THC (where legal) can be rubbed into the skin of the abdomen or onto the lower back with varying degrees of success. No studies exist to guide the dosing. I have recommended topicals to my patients who wished to try something low-risk, and some have reported it has made a difference. The effect likely depends on the type of topical used and also the other ingredients, but in theory it may have a localised anti-inflammatory effect depending on how well absorbed it is (but again no published studies exist to prove this). This is a very safe way to use THC for period pain, as topicals with THC generally do not make you feel high or cause impairment (unless they are transdermal patches they do not absorb systemically it seems), and if they offer relief, they may be a welcome addition to your toolkit.

PMS and PMDD

PMS (premenstrual syndrome) is a combination of symptoms experienced by up to 90% of women to some degree about a week or two before their period (the first day of bleeding). The symptoms can include bloating, mood shifts, headaches, irritability and feelings of stress and fatigue, and can range from the mild to the severe. PMDD (premenstrual dysmorphic disorder) is a severe form of PMS involving more severe mood changes, including depression, anxiety and mood swings the week before the first day of your period, with the symptoms improving once your period has started.

Our own endocannabinoid AEA peaks around ovulation, so it is possible that PMS symptoms in the second half of the menstrual cycle may be related to falling endocannabinoid levels. A study showed that women who suffer with depression have lower levels of 2-AG, one of our main endocannabinoids (see Chapter Four). Symptoms of low mood, anxiety or irritability, in addition to being related to our other hormone fluctuations in the second half of our cycle, may also be related to these endocannabinoid levels. This may explain why inhaled or oral cannabis in the premenstrual phase (which is around one week before the start of your period) can help with PMS mood and other symptoms in many women.

Cara's story

Cara came to see me for anxiety and PMDD. She was already taking an SSRI mood medication, which was having sexual side effects and made her feel flat emotionally, and trying to do yoga and meditate, but it just wasn't enough for that week before her period. She had recently come off the Pill after many years, and had felt her PMDD return full force. She really wanted to try something more natural but was afraid of taking THC cannabis, because as a teen she had smoked cannabis a few times and had a severe anxiety reaction, which she did not want to repeat.

We decided to try a high-CBD product with minimal THC. I prescribed a very high-CBD, low-THC oil every day, and we upped the dose the week before Cara's period. After three menstrual cycles she saw a huge difference in her mood. This led her to reduce her SSRI pills to the lowest possible dose, which meant the side effects disappeared. Cara was so grateful for the change. Knowing she no longer had to dread and fear the last week of her cycle each month had led to massively positive changes in her relationship and self-confidence.

How to use CBD for PMS and PMDD

To help balance mood and irritability across the whole cycle, adding a CBD oil daily is a good way to start, using the general dose of 10 mg 3x/day with meals and increasing gradually as needed, keeping in mind that everyone is slightly different. If you suffer with some degree of anxiety or stress/burnout all month long, I recommend this option (see Chapters Eight and Nine). Alternatively, you can try using it for just the second half of your cycle (i.e. day 14, when you ovulate, to the first day of your period) if your symptoms are experienced only in the week or so before your first day of bleeding. If just using for this half of the cycle, start at a higher dose of 15–20 mg 3x/day with meals and go up as needed. You can experiment with one of these options for at least three cycles and see what changes you notice.

PROBLEMS COMING OFF THE PILL

Many women experience what Yale medical doctor and women's health advocate Dr Aviva Romm calls post-Pill syndrome. Although this is not technically a medical diagnosis, it refers to when your cycle doesn't return to normal for three to six months after stopping the Pill. This can mean heavy or painful periods, irregular periods, bloating, moodiness or acne, or any combination of these. The reason usually is down to the Pill just covering up these issues for years, and when you remove it – bam! The problem is back again and often worse than before. Some experts also feel that in some women, there may be a post-Pill communication issue between the hypothalamus (which controls cycles) and the ovaries. While I don't believe cannabis is a cure-all for this issue, CBD, and sometimes medical cannabis, can help in the transition period coming off the Pill with symptoms like PMS and period pain. It may also help with acne when used topically with skincare. In any case it is very important to get to the bottom of what is causing the returned issues, and rule out conditions such as PCOS (polycystic ovary syndrome) or low thyroid.

Endometriosis

Endometriosis is an extremely painful condition where the lining of the uterus grows outside the womb. The exact relationship between the endocannabinoid system and endometriosis is still not totally understood. One study that looked at women with endometriosis found that they had differences in cannabinoid receptors in the endometrial tissue sampled when compared to women without the condition. This suggests that the ECS does indeed play a role in endometriosis.[9]

Preliminary research appears to suggest that plant cannabinoids such as THC (and possibly, via inflammation pathways, CBD) may help reduce pain from endometriosis.[10, 11] A study in Australia looked at cannabis as part of a self-treatment approach to endometriosis. In that study, patients found it was more effective than the use of heat, exercise, rest, breathing or meditation exercises, or any physical activity such as yoga or stretching. These are findings that we cannot ignore or write off as chance or placebo, and are very promising since the pain from this disease is often debilitating for many women.

However, the story gets a bit more complicated from here, thanks to some *in vitro* (test tube) non-human studies that suggest THC may induce migration of tissue outside of the womb,[12] which in plain English means that it may spread endometriosis further, possibly making it worse. This was only demonstrated in a Petri dish, not in a human body, so it doesn't mean it will work the same in us, but it's a caution that highlights how much we still don't know. Another study using animal models found that activating the CB1 receptor with a synthetic drug[13] seems to promote the spreading of endometriosis (i.e. makes it worse), but we don't know how exactly that applies to plant cannabinoids or if it translates in humans.

In summary, cannabis seems promising for endometriosis pain, but the effect on the disease itself is still unsure and we need more studies to tease it all out. If you do want to use cannabis for symptom control, you can start by trying a daily CBD oil from hemp, starting at 10 mg 3x/day and increasing the dose every few days or every week. The optimal dose is unknown, but generally if you reach a dose of between 60 and 80 mg/day, stay here for a few months at least to see if there will be a gradual perceived symptom benefit over time.

On the medical cannabis side, it seems safest to start by trying a high-CBD, low-THC strain for both oils and vaporised cannabis since THC may contribute to a possible downside in endometriosis. However, this downside must be weighed against the upside of a small dose of THC. Even a micro dose of 2 mg can help immensely with pain relief and improve quality of life.

Fertility

The exact effect of cannabis, and even hemp CBD wellness products, on female fertility is still being researched, and so far we only have preliminary data and one human study on healthy women to go by. On a population level, groups of women such as the followers of the Rastafarian religion in Jamaica regularly consume cannabis, often in the form of tea or edibles, and there has been no reported evidence of decreased fertility rates in this group compared to the general population. However, the evidence is sparse on the topic of cannabis and fertility more generally. So far, most studies are looking at the pregnancy and post-natal effects on infants (see pp.237–40 below).[14]

Other studies on the effects of chronic cannabis use on fertility have been mixed. In some, the results suggest that regular cannabis use may lead to a shortened luteal phase (the second phase of the menstrual cycle, leading up to the period) and in one study that women may have a higher chance of delayed ovulation, although in other studies no such difference was found.[15, 16] In short, the research is still very early for conclusive evidence.[17] A short luteal phase may not in itself be an issue or a cause of decreased fertility as long as other hormone levels are normal and ovulation is happening, so it is unclear if this possible cannabis effect is something clinically important and how much it may affect fertility[18]

In animals, chronic cannabis exposure led to a disruption of menstrual cycles and ovulation in female rats, as well as changed levels of sex hormone such as LH (luteinising hormone), which is important for ovulation and fertility.[19] So far it seems that an important factor in how cannabis affects our cycles is the amount of cannabis, and THC in particular, that is consumed regularly.

Lastly, one large study looked at couples trying to become pregnant, and their self-reported cannabis use habits, and found there was no association between cannabis use (even frequent use) and the time it took to become pregnant.[20] This was not a controlled study, which many will point out, correctly, as a major drawback. However, it is still some level of evidence, albeit a preliminary one, that cannabis may not have a major effect on fertility in normally fertile women and men.

According to the published research available so far, it seems the effects of plant cannabinoids on the ovarian and period hormones are likely dose-dependent and may also depend on individual differences. This is the case with the effects of cannabis on most other body systems too. Lower-THC, higher-CBD low-dose cannabis therapy may be relatively safe and is of course very different to self-medicating with high-THC cannabis without medical supervision. But the reality is we just don't know for sure yet. So many factors can affect fertility, it is hard to pin down the effects of cannabis and tease them out from everything else.

For an integrative medicine doctor who tries to look at the full picture, the confusing information we have so far highlights the fact that any intervention – even taking something natural – can have real effects on us and our hormone cycles. So it's always wise to be cautious and not just assume something is totally safe and without risk just because it comes from a plant. A good example of this is the innocuous-sounding liquorice tea. I have known multiple newly pregnant friends (and a few new patients who were already pregnant) to still consume liquorice tea (or in a supplement form for stress), believing it was safe and natural. They had no idea liquorice tea is considered a huge no-no during pregnancy, even though the risk is likely a very small one. It may increase the possibility of early pregnancy loss (spontaneous abortion) due to the oestrogen-mimicking effects of the active ingredient, glycyrrhizin. When I find out, I tell them to stop drinking it immediately and try not to overly panic them. So far I have not seen any bad outcomes personally that were attributable to the liquorice tea intake, but it is best to be careful.

Based on where we are at currently with our knowledge about cannabis and fertility, if a woman is healthy and has no need for cannabis medicines, it is generally advised to avoid cannabis (i.e. recreational use!) if you are actively trying to become pregnant, especially if:

- You are new(ish) to THC. Chronic users, at least in theory, may have adapted their hormone levels to this new 'steady state' at least in theory if they have been consuming cannabis with THC daily or nearly daily for years.

- You have been told by your doctor that you have (or may have) fertility issues.
- You are aged 35 or over and actively trying to conceive, since our fertility naturally decreases as we age.

The advice on what to do about CBD wellness products from hemp is less clear as far as studies go (i.e. there are none!), but there is no evidence that using CBD decreases fertility. All studies so far, even in animals, have been on cannabis containing significant THC. Hemp-based CBD products are already being used effectively for other conditions that may affect fertility and health,[21] such as anxiety, burnout, toxic stress, chronic fatigue (which can also cause high stress hormone and lower progesterone, therefore disrupting female hormones) and pain. So CBD may be of less risk than the drugs it replaced, which often have an unknown effect at best on fertility.

I always remind both my patients and colleagues that stress itself decreases fertility by stealing our progesterone and increasing cortisol (stress hormone) and is the number one cause of idiopathic (non-anatomical) infertility and lack of ovulation. I have had many patients over the years who were investigated for infertility and no cause could be found. After getting them on a daily mind-body routine for stress (and sometimes supplements), as well as implementing lifestyle changes, they became pregnant naturally without needing IVF or other intervention.

Pregnancy and breastfeeding

The ECS regulates almost every part of female reproduction, from producing eggs for future fertilisation through implantation of a embryo and all the way to giving birth and the post-partum period.[22]

One study done in a test tube (so again, not in humans) showed that cannabis affected the crosstalk between cells[23] that create the nutrient-rich environment in the womb to support the placenta and very early-stage embryo, while another test-tube study suggests that THC may negatively impact the growth of the placenta cells,[24] but these findings have not yet been proven to happen inside an actual uterus in humans. So it's only speculation what this actually means for us and, if it is an issue, how much cannabis would have to be consumed for it to be detrimental to an early pregnancy.

Anything that suppresses LH (luteinising hormone) during the early second half of our cycle right after ovulation may potentially contribute to an early pregnancy loss by reducing another key hormone, progesterone,[25] that is needed to maintain and support a pregnancy. A study in rhesus monkeys found that a single large injected dose of THC during this important phase of the menstrual cycle decreased circulating progesterone levels.

Whether cannabis can actually cause a pregnancy loss at the usual doses consumed is still up for debate, but as with any substance in pregnancy, avoidance and caution is the best approach when there are question marks. We do know that THC crosses the placenta to have a possible effect on the developing infant.[26] While it is true that there is still limited evidence that maternal cannabis use (mostly from smoked cannabis) can cause pregnancy complications, there is some evidence that cannabis (we think mainly high-THC forms) may be a risk factor for a lower-birth-weight baby.

What about cannabis and developmental issues in babies when mothers use it while pregnant? Apart from lower birth weights, another question is if a child develops problems later on that can be traced back to cannabis exposure in the womb. The answer is we don't know for sure yet that exposure to THC-containing cannabis has a lasting effect. There is conflicting evidence for a link between cannabis exposure in the womb and neurocognitive function (cognitive and behavioural differences) when compared to children with no exposure to cannabis. What this means is that some studies show no link, while others show a possible positive link between cannabis exposure and neurocognitive function.[27] So until more is known about the possible effects in both the short and long term for the baby, and whether there is a safe limit of cannabis (and THC especially) while pregnant (currently this is also unknown), it is best to avoid cannabis use in pregnancy and while breastfeeding, or at the very least keep the THC to a minimum for harm reduction.[28]

Although I do not prescribe medical cannabis in pregnancy nor recommend it for pregnant women, I have had a few patients continue to use high-CBD, low-THC cannabis in oral oil form from a dispensary while pregnant (against my medical advice) to control their anxiety disorder and insomnia. These patients decided that even with this possible risk and against my official medical advice, it was preferable to going back on other anti-anxiety drugs that also may carry a risk that they considered similar. And of course there is a risk in taking no treatment for their anxiety and what effect that may have on their pregnancy and developing child. No pregnancy or labour complications resulted in these patients. The children are still infants and toddlers but so far appear to have normal development, and the mothers were able to get through their pregnancy and post-partum periods with ease, which is not always the case if you suffer with an anxiety or sleep disorder.

So it's not always clear-cut, and what is best for one woman may not be best for another. If, after speaking with your doctor, you decide together that the benefits outweigh the possible risks, I still recommend sticking to low-dose and low-THC products or CBD hemp products from a reputable non-contaminated and lab-tested source to reduce possible or potential unknown risks. There are currently no published studies on hemp-based CBD wellness products in pregnancy, as all the data so far (and there isn't very much) has focused on THC-containing cannabis. They are probably relatively harmless, especially at low doses, but until we have studies to prove this, there is still a giant blank in terms of our definite knowledge about their possible effects on pregnancy and the breastfeeding baby. We are unlikely to ever get these studies, as testing products in pregnancy and breastfeeding is understandably a minefield, even if you can get approval to conduct the study in the first place. So just like other herbs and drugs where we don't know, avoidance is probably safest for healthy women except in cases where CBD is thought to have enough benefits to justify the unknown risks.

Hyperemesis gravidarum

The same goes with my advice with hyperemesis gravidarum – severe persistent nausea and vomiting during pregnancy. This condition can threaten the pregnancy if it is serious enough to cause weight loss or malnutrition and require hospitalisation. Some experts believe a low dose of a balanced (1:1 CBD to THC) cannabis product via inhalation has a favourable risk–benefit ratio in these cases. This may be especially true where other drug options may also carry a risk,[29] especially if the first-line recommended drugs that have good safety data aren't enough. The problem is that collecting data is hard because even if women are self-medicating with cannabis for this issue, they are often afraid to disclose this information due to the stigma (and in many cases cannabis being illegal in that area without a prescription).[30] Cannabis has been used traditionally to treat nausea for hundreds of years. However, I still recommend trying the first-line drug and non-drug approaches first and discussing the pros and cons with your pregnancy doctor to find what is best for you in this situation.

Perimenopausal and menopausal symptoms

Menopause is defined as no menstrual cycle for 12 months, and the perimenopausal years are the lead-up to this eventual shift. Symptoms of menopause generally start in perimenopause and can include hot flashes, night sweats, vaginal dryness, mood swings, irritability, loss of libido, bloating, frequent urination, weight gain and memory lapses. For some, these symptoms are mild, while for others they are severe and crippling, capable of ruining their life if they try to go it alone. Many of my patients describe their perimenopausal and menopause years as feeling like an imposter hijacked their brain, because they just didn't feel like themselves. Thankfully, there is much you can do to help make this natural transition more smoothly and with fewer problematic symptoms. One of these tools is cannabis and CBD.

The good thing about treating menopausal symptoms with

cannabis is that any issue around possible effects on fertility or cycle length are no longer a concern. The main goal is getting control over hot flashes, poor sleep, irritability, fatigue and brain fog. I have had many women come to see me who did not want to try HRT (hormone replacement therapy) and had already tried the other recommended conventional treatments like antidepressants and anti-anxiety medications as well as sleeping tablets. They wished to try a more natural approach, understanding that it was not standard care or considered a first-line therapy. In addition to experiencing menopausal symptoms, they all had another issue going on too: insomnia (even before the menopause), anxiety, chronic pain, fibromyalgia and restless legs just to name a few. So for them, medical cannabis was doing double duty, as is often the case in most of my patients.

The reasons why CBD oil from hemp as well as THC-containing cannabis may help support perimenopause wellness are probably numerous. CBD, for example, acts on our serotonin system (which helps balance our mood – think of it as our happy hormone) as well as on anti-inflammatory pathways. THC is also an anti-inflammatory neuroprotective chemical that can help regulate sleep cycles if they are dysfunctional and assist with pain of many varieties. These are all issues that can arise in perimenopause. Perhaps unsurprisingly, given what we know about medical research and the female body, there is almost no published data on cannabis for menopausal symptoms, despite the many patients and clients who have self-treated successfully. The only study I found on an extensive hunt on the topic was a small one polling women who used cannabis to help with symptoms such as joint/muscle aches, irritability, sleep problems, depression, anxiety and hot flashes.[31] The researchers concluded that, given our ageing population, we should probably investigate the potential of medical cannabis as a valid treatment for these symptoms (duh!). When it comes to sleep disruption and night-time symptoms in the perimenopause phase, one contributor seems to be reduced levels of GABA, our calming neurotransmitter. Adding plant cannabinoids may help modulate (i.e. make normal again) GABA levels. More GABA seems to equal a calmer brain and more restful sleep.

Carol's story

Carol came to see me for a constellation of anxiety, fibromyalgia and sleeping issues. When we sat down together for the first time, however, it was her menopausal symptoms that were driving her crazy and making her other already overlapping issues much worse. She had a strong family history of breast cancer so didn't want to go on HRT. She had already cut out sugar and alcohol but was still at the end of her rope with her feelings of irritability and being overwhelmed by what she described as 'the slightest thing'. This had resulted in some major arguments with her husband and friends. She said it felt like an alien had taken control of her personality some days.

We decided to try cannabis along with a mindfulness practice, a sleep reset plan using non-drug approaches and some other natural safe supplements to help with her menopausal symptoms. We chose a very high-CBD, low-THC oil for the daytime and a small dose of a THC-dominant oil for her night restlessness and sleep disturbance. On the occasional day where she felt foggy and fatigued, we added a small amount of balanced (1:1 CBD to THC ratio) vaporised cannabis and for the evenings, to help with anxiety and irritability, an indica-labelled calming strain as needed. She found she only used these a few times a week, very sparingly, but they allowed her to discontinue the daily benzodiazepine pills she was needing for rescue and she had no side effects from the cannabis. Three months later, she said she felt like a new person; she was sleeping better, had more energy and felt less foggy and irritable. All in all, it was a huge success and really changed her quality of life and helped ease her transition through the menopause.

How to use CBD wellness products (hemp CBD) for menopausal symptoms

- Try a full-spectrum or broad-spectrum CBD oil.
- Look for terpenes that are calming, mood-balancing and anti-inflammatory (check the label):
    - beta-caryophyllene – anti-inflammatory, also in black pepper

- linalool – smells flowery, like lavender
- myrcene – smells earthy/peppery, like hops, and is one of the most common terpenes
- terpinolene – smells fresh, like a mix of flowers and pine
- D-limonene – smells like lemons and has both anti-anxiety and antidepressant effects, so is thought of as a mood-balancing terpene.

Starting dose and titrating up

Try starting with 10 mg of CBD first thing in the morning, at midday/early afternoon (12–2 p.m.) and at dinner time for a total of 30 mg/day. Stay at this dose for a few days to a week or so and track your symptoms to test how you feel:

- Identify your main symptoms. Are they improving?
- Are they still bad at a certain time of day (e.g. worse in the evening)?
- Are you still having trouble getting to sleep or staying asleep?

Remember: there is no specific perfect dose that works for everyone exactly the same, especially since menopause symptoms can vary widely and each person's endocannabinoid system balance is unique, so self-titration is the name of the game. Everyone may be a bit different as to what dose may be best for them, and this optimal dose may change as hormone levels continue to alter over months.

Non-cannabis helpers to add

In addition to CBD, I also use specific botanicals and lifestyle changes to help with symptoms of menopause.

- For stress reduction and enhancing brain flexibility:
  - mindfulness meditation – helps with irritability and mood changes and lowers cortisol (increased cortisol makes

hormone imbalances worse in the perimenopausal phase, which leads to worse symptoms)

- yoga or t'ai chi – helps stabilise and calm the fight-or-flight response and overactivity in favour of the rest-and-digest arm of the nervous system, as well as reduce cortisol and enhance cognition.
- Hormone-balancing diet:
  - rich in plant-based foods and veggies
  - whole grains only; cut out the 'whites': white bread, pastries, flour, crackers, pizza, regular pasta, bagels, baked goods, white rice
  - low glycaemic index (high-sugar foods increase weight gain, insulin resistance and inflammation)
  - all meat should be organic, grass-fed (red meat) and hormone-free
  - gluten-free – gluten grains can inhibit CYP 450 enzymes, which may contribute to increased oestrogen dominance and further hormonal imbalances, so stick to eating non-gluten grains such as brown rice, wild rice, quinoa, millet, buckwheat, teff
  - cut out all alcohol for a trial period of eight weeks; if you do add it back in after that, keep it to one serving (a small glass of wine or less/day).
- Menopause botanicals: chasteberry, liquorice, passionflower, reishi mushrooms, maca, Estrovera (a supplement with the active ingredient called ERr 731, a special extract of rhubarb root).
- Swap coffee for herbal tulsi (holy basil) tea for a more natural energy, as caffeine may make your anxiety worse and deplete magnesium.
- Natural supplements: magnesium, B6 and B complex, vitamin D, zinc if depression/low moods are an issue (see Chapter Ten).
- Sleep support (see Chapter Eleven).
- Quit cigarette smoking – studies show smokers have worse menopausal symptoms than non-smokers.

How to use medical cannabis products for general menopausal symptoms

Only try this under the supervision of a doctor and, of course, if medical cannabis (containing THC) is legal where you live. This advice is for general symptoms, but if you wish to target specific symptoms, such as anxiety, stress/burnout/fatigue, sleep or pain, please see individual chapters for details.

- Start with a high-CBD cannabis oil as your base, taken orally.
- Average starting dose: 5–10 mg 3x/day, taken with meals, for a total of 30 mg. The THC dose will depend on the product, but start with 1–2 mg of daytime THC max. (i.e. an oil that has a THC to CBD ratio of 1:10 will give you 1 mg of THC for every 10 mg of CBD). THC micro-dosing along with CBD can benefit menopausal symptoms in many women.
- Stay at this dose for 1–2 weeks and use a symptom tracker or journal to rate and track how you feel.
- Keep increasing the dose until you feel the symptoms improving.
- For sleep problems, try an additional 2 mg dose of THC using a THC oil labelled as 'indica' and high in myrcene and CBN (see Chapter Eleven).
- Choose strains high in CBD and low in THC to start with (a good ratio of CBD to THC is between 10:1 and 20:1, meaning between 10 and 20 parts CBD to every 1 part THC).

Using vaporising cannabis flowers for menopausal symptoms

For reducing anxiety, fatigue, irritability and stress that comes on suddenly, vaporised cannabis can give a faster result and also wear off faster as opposed to an oral oil.

- Start with high-CBD, low-THC flowers, especially if you have never had THC before (a ratio of 10:1 CBD to THC or higher).

- If this has no effect, you can try a balanced strain with equal amounts of CBD and THC (i.e. 1:1).
- Start with a matchstick-head-sized amount, especially if it is a strain with more THC (i.e. a balanced strain).
- Some women find this helpful to get them in the right state of mind to practise mindfulness meditation or yoga.
- Can often be used as a replacement for anxiety pills such as benzodiazepines which are weaned down on slowly with your doctor under medical supervision.
- Cannabis flower can also be used before bedtime to help you get to sleep more easily and wind down a busy mind, using a traditionally labelled sedating 'indica or broad-leaf ' strain high in myrcene (see Chapter Eleven for details).
- For additional details of how to use cannabis for a specific troublesome symptom, refer to the relevant chapter.

Fibroids

Fibroids are benign (non-cancerous) tumours or growths in the uterus that, if they reach a big enough size, can cause many problematic symptoms. The exact cause of fibroids is not well understood, but multiple factors including genetics, dietary choices, gut health, environmental toxins, stress and problems getting rid of excess oestrogen from the body are thought to contribute to them. They can cause very heavy periods, iron deficiency, painful periods, bloating and discomfort, especially if they continue to grow in size. An integrative medicine approach includes a diet high in oestrogen-detoxifying foods (cruciferous veggies) that is also low in sugar and gluten-free. It also includes supplements, herbals and exercise as well as things like acupuncture and bioidentical hormones if needed. This is not a cure but can be helpful in managing fibroids using the best of East and West.

This is another area that deserves more research, since we know that the ECS may play a role in fibroids. One study showed that in people with fibroids the ECS balance was off; specifically, the CB1 to CB2 cannabinoid receptor ratio was lower than normal. This may suggest that this imbalance could be a possible treatment target for new cannabinoid-derived drugs. It is unclear how plant cannabinoids may play a role, however. Hopefully we will discover more soon, given that the current treatment options for fibroids are limited, as are their long-term effectiveness.[32] CBD, however, may reduce stress, and multiple recent studies have demonstrated a link between stress and risk of fibroids, as well as fibroid symptom severity.[33, 34] So adding a daily CBD oil may be helpful indirectly as part of a holistic approach if you suffer with fibroids (see Chapter Eight).

I also approach problems like fibroids with additional holistic approaches, which do not cure the issue but may help reduce some of the complex underlying factors. These approaches include helping restore healthy gut bacteria through diet and probiotics, as well as healthy fibre; avoiding environmental toxins such as pesticides and herbicides (e.g. avoiding heavily sprayed fruits and vegetables); cutting out dairy and other inflammatory foods; and supplementing with 2000 IU of vitamin D each day (since low vitamin D levels are linked to fibroids, and in northern hemisphere countries like the UK, many people are deficient without knowing it).

PCOS

PCOS (polycystic ovary syndrome) is a hormone imbalance disorder affecting up to 15% of women of reproductive age.[35] It has three main features:

- irregular periods and lack of regular ovulation
- excess androgens (male hormones), which can cause acne and increased facial hair
- fluid-filled sacs called cysts on one or both ovaries

It is also associated with abnormal blood sugar control and insulin regulation (insulin resistance), and problems with not being able to lose weight.

We know that dysfunction within the endocannabinoid system seems to play a role in PCOS, and that THC from cannabis may activate the CB1 receptors, possibly decrease progesterone and increase the oestrogen imbalance problem. So in general, until we know more it is best to avoid THC if you have PCOS, unless there is some other reason or condition where it may be indicated and where the possible downside may be overshadowed by the potential benefit. This is not a call to make alone; it is something a doctor trained in this area can help you assess so that you can make a decision together.

CBD wellness products, meaning hemp-based CBD oil or other products like patches etc, may help with metabolic issues like insulin resistance in some people. There have been no big studies to prove the link, but I have seen many patients on high-CBD, low-THC cannabis oil who had improved insulin resistance and blood sugar control six months after starting it with no other major lifestyle changes. That clinical experience suggests that taking a CBD oil for general wellness may be beneficial indirectly for PCOS, by helping with insulin resistance, as has been shown in studies on rats with diabetes[36] and insulin resistance metabolic dysfunction[37] (pre-diabetes), and also with losing weight.[38] Combining CBD with THCV, a minor cannabinoid, may enhance the beneficial effect on insulin resistance.[39]

For additional information, see reference[40].

CHAPTER FOURTEEN

ENHANCING SEX AND LIBIDO

Who doesn't want to have better sex? Whether it's solo sex and self-pleasuring, or sex with a partner (or both!), the desire for sex and intimacy is a basic human driver. However, despite its great importance, thanks to the hectic pace and stresses of modern life and just everyday scheduling challenges, making time for sex and getting back into the groove after you've been in a sexual slump can be tricky. Any tool that can help is usually of great curiosity no matter what your age, gender or orientation may be.

In the US, where cannabis has been legalised for both medical and recreational purposes in many states, people who use cannabis have 20% more sex than everyone else, after adjusting for things like age, according to a study from Stanford University.[1] A third of US women have tried cannabis for sex, reporting that it helps them have more satisfying orgasms. In places where cannabis with THC is not yet legal without a medical prescription (and convincing your doctor to give it to you for improving your sex life may be a bit of a stretch!), there is still CBD, which may not be quite as exciting (or potent for feeling more in the mood) but is a very safe way to dip your toe in the water of combining a cannabis plant product with getting frisky.

When it comes to cannabis and sex, the two have a long history together. Cannabis has been used since ancient times to both stimulate libido, or sexual desire, and purposely inhibit the desire for sex. Much like with anxiety and other uses, with THC at least the result seems to be dose-dependent. At low and even micro doses, many studies report that THC enhances the sexual experience from many angles: desire, sensation, orgasm and relaxation around the sexual experience to fully savour the moment and experience. At high doses, performance and desire can both be negatively affected. The cannabis and sex (and THC) sweet spot changes from person to person because – as you probably know by now if you have read this far in the book – everyone's endocannabinoid system (and hormone system that influences all things to do with sex!) balance is a bit unique. Even the same person can change their system's balance depending on current stress levels and other life factors.

Bob's story

Bob came to see me as a patient with his wife, Cheryl. Bob suffered with chronic back pain and wanted to know if cannabis could help. He and Cheryl had been married for almost 10 years, and overall they had a great relationship. However, due to work schedules, stresses and his chronic pain, they had rarely had the desire to have sex over the past few years.

Although the main medical reason for referral was chronic pain, as we worked together and added medical cannabis to his pain treatment, Bob also noticed the positive effect a bit of vaporised cannabis had on his sex life. At his follow-up visit, he said that in addition to helping take the edge off the pain, it had also led to him and Cheryl rekindling their romantic and sexual relationship – an unexpected perk! It helped him feel more in the mood and enjoy sex more. Although his chronic back pain was the main source of pain overall, he also had a feeling of tightness and discomfort in his pelvis, and the cannabis seemed to help with this too, especially during sex and intimate play. It was a positive cycle, because once he started initiating more sex, it boosted his sexual confidence and Cheryl also became more interested again. As a couple, they went from sex feeling slightly stressful and pressured and 'a bit of a chore' to pleasurable and unforced. The performance anxiety they both felt because sex had been strained for so long was massively helped by a little bit of vaporised cannabis. Bob said it was like when they were newlyweds, only better!

How cannabis and CBD may make sex better

Cannabis products can set the stage for better, more enjoyable sex and sensual play by helping relieve 'flow blockers' to feeling sexy, such as anxiety, stress, fatigue and pain. The right strains can also help boost mood. I always tell patients too that sex doesn't have to mean intercourse, or even any form of penetration; it includes all sorts of play that may be more enjoyable for the parties involved. For example, if one partner suffers from pelvic pain (which can affect both women and men) or vulvodynia (in women, where even gentle contact can cause pain or discomfort), cannabis topicals may help make sensual play and touch more enjoyable, based on many women's self-reporting. Although currently there are no studies to support this directly – cannabis and sexual function is still a new frontier – research has begun, with one recent study showing that THC reduced induced-vulvodynia symptoms in an animal model.[2] If you are trying to conceive, intercourse is obviously the main course on the sex menu, but outside of that scenario, cannabis can help you get creative about sex and start thinking of it in broader terms, which can shake things up and enhance pleasure in itself.

Combining cannabis with sex, especially at certain times in a woman's cycle (around mid-cycle, the time of ovulation), may help increase the chance of having an orgasm. If that is already easy for you on any day of the month (lucky you!), it may also help enhance the quality of your orgasm. This is based on many self-report studies that polled women about what effect cannabis has on sex for them in terms of sexual experience quality as well as orgasm strength. It's also all about the type of cannabis, the dose and especially the amount of THC consumed, since too much THC can make orgasm harder to achieve, at least in men.

Forget wine and Viagra; try some cannabis!

When people want to get in the mood or spice things up, the substance of choice for foreplay is most often wine or other alcohol. This doesn't, however, work well for everyone. From personal experience as well as that of many of my friends, patients and clients, alcohol doesn't always make us feel super-sexy – we can even end up feeling more sluggish or tired, especially after a long day. For many people, cannabis is a better substance to mix with foreplay and sex. Even CBD mocktails followed by a massage with intimate-parts-friendly CBD massage oil can do the trick for many people who want a healthier alternative helper to getting friskier. Cannabis sexual health products have the potential to be the new Viagra and, in fact, some of the same researchers who developed that drug are now working on cannabinoids for sexual performance. Many men who have previously used Viagra as a sex aid also tell me they now prefer the experience of using cannabis, due to the more subtle effects (at low doses) and the increase in sensation, as well as the enhanced feeling of connection with a partner that they don't get with Viagra or similar drugs.

How our endocannabinoid system gets in on the big 'O' moment

Research studies have shown that right after an orgasm, we release a burst of natural endocannabinoids.[3] This may account for part of the 'post-O glow' period both men and women experience. Healthy endocannabinoid system function (as well as the use of plant cannabinoids) can also help take the nervous system out of fight-or-flight (sympathetic) mode and into rest-and-digest (parasympathetic) mode. This is because cannabinoids act on the amygdala and the hypothalamus, two of the brain areas involved in sexual function and sex behaviour. CB1 receptor activation can also delay the time to orgasm – something THC may do too. That may be helpful if one suffers with premature ejaculation, but if not, an excess of THC may delay orgasm too much.[4] Again, it's about finding the personalised cannabis–sex sweet spot unique to you.

What about sperm count and cannabis in men? This is a question I often get asked by patients. In animal models, cannabis decreases sperm count.[5] However, this has not been proven in humans. If it is the case, it is likely to be a dose-dependent effect and likely with THC in particular. However, couples trying to conceive should be aware of this potential (especially for high-THC cannabis) until we know more.[6]

Hemp-based CBD products for sex

CBD products made from hemp are a good option if you are keen to introduce a cannabis plant product into your sex life but want to avoid THC, or if THC products are not legally available where you live. CBD taken by mouth (as an oil or in capsules) or via a sublingual spray or a transdermal patch may help reduce tension, stress and anxiety and even some forms of pain (see individual chapters for each of these issues). That in itself is enough to light a spark in your sex life if it relieves issues that cause you to feel anything but in the mood. Then there are the CBD topicals: lubes, intimate massage oils and the like. The vulva mucosa and clitoris skin in women and the scrotal and penile skin in men is more porous than non-genital skin, possibly allowing greater absorption, so if there is irritation or inflammation in these areas contributing to discomfort with sex, it is possible that CBD may be helpful for some people as an ingredient in a lubricant. Currently there are no published research studies on the sexually enhancing effects of these products, but there are women (I've met them!) who claim they have made a difference for them.

Taking hemp-based CBD by mouth

CBD oils or sublingual tinctures may not lead to the immediately noticeable effect experienced with THC products; however, a dose of say 30–60 mg of CBD taken 30–60 minutes before sex may make some people feel more relaxed and in the mood. This result is self-reported by my patients, friends and clients (and is something I find useful myself as well!), although no published studies exist yet to guide on this specific point of use. Smaller doses may have an effect for some people too (everyone is a bit different), but even high doses are very safe to try; just experiment with what you find does the trick for you.

Vaporising hemp-based CBD

In some places in the EU such as Switzerland, you can find what is called CBD flower, which contains less than 0.2% THC but smells and looks like normal weed or cannabis dried flower. This is also sold on the grey market in the UK and by some shops, although it is not officially a legal product at the time of writing due to a legal technicality. However, it is quite safe as long as it is from a reputable source and contains no contaminants, just like any other form of CBD. CBD flower can be inhaled to get CBD into the bloodstream more quickly and in higher amounts than oils or sublingual forms. Start with a few matchstick-head-sized pieces (see Chapter Five for details of all things vaporising). Take 1–3 inhalations, then wait 5 minutes or so and see how you feel. You can put new flower in and repeat, since CBD flower is almost impossible to overdose on. It only contains trace THC, so it won't get you high, but it may make you feel more relaxed.

CBD topicals

First off, if you are using condoms (which is the best way to prevent STIs and also the best barrier method for avoiding pregnancy), never use *any* oil-based personal lubricants or massage oils as the oil can cause them to break down and fail. That includes any natural lubricant like coconut oil or sesame oil. Generally, only water-based lubricants that state that they can be used safely with condoms are OK.

CBD lubes, including oil-based ones, are generally considered safe to use with a high-quality silicone sex toy like a vibrator or dildo, as they will not break down the silicone in the toy.

A good lubricant in general, even without CBD, can help with comfort during sexual play and intercourse by reducing friction and discomfort. This is especially true if the natural vaginal lubrication is decreased, which happens naturally as women age and enter perimenopause and menopause, due to hormone shifts and decrease in oestrogen. If this is an issue for you, do ask your doctor about bioidentical hormones used topically for severe atrophy/bleeding.

If you are sensitive to yeast infections, UTIs (bladder infections) and the like, I recommend choosing a pH-balanced product without potentially irritating ingredients. Just because the product contains natural CBD doesn't automatically make it non-irritating! These are some other ingredients to avoid in all topical lubes:

- Glycerine or glycerol and propylene glycol. Often found in water-based lubes, these may be a food source for yeast (so increased chance of a yeast infection) and can also be an irritant for some women. The WHO recommends total glycerol content less than 8.3%.
- Parabens. These preservatives may act as what are known as endocrine disruptors, which may disrupt hormones.
- Chlorhexidine and derivatives. This preservative in some lubes is a topical antiseptic, so can kill the healthy normal vaginal bacteria that protect against infections.
- Polyquaternium. The WHO suggests avoiding this ingredient as it may increase the chance of HIV virus transmission from an infected partner.
- Hydroxyethylcellulose. This is made from plant fibre and creates the gliding, slippery effect of some lubes. Generally this one is not an issue for many people, but if you get frequent or recurrent yeast infections you may want to choose a lube without it, as it may feed the yeast.
- Petroleum jelly (Vaseline). I can tell you from running women's health clinics that using petroleum jelly as a lubricant is not a good idea. I have treated many women experiencing bacterial vaginosis or a severe yeast infection with copious discharge after sex using petroleum jelly,[7] and multiple studies have proven this is a real thing.
- If you are trying to get pregnant, you might want to avoid olive oil as a base, because one study found it may have a negative effect on sperm,[8] although unless there is a fertility issue with either partner, this effect may be minimal.

THC-containing cannabis products for sex

Everyone reacts slightly differently to cannabis when it comes to sex, although in general most people find a very small dose of THC positive. The first and most obvious use for a cannabis product containing THC is helping reduce any chronic pain that could be impeding sexual enjoyment. This includes chronic pelvic pain, which affects both men and women and is often unrecognised (no one asks the patient about it) and under-diagnosed, especially in men. Cannabis by oral routes (oils, sprays, capsules) and vaporised cannabis are now considered valid options for dealing with chronic pelvic pain by mainstream medicine bodies, including some urologists who specialise in this area.[9] If reducing any sort of chronic pain is the main goal for you, see Chapter Twelve.

As with every use of cannabis, depending on the mode of use, the THC content and the strain, the effects can still vary from person to person. For example, if you vaporise a strain labelled as 'indica' with lots of that myrcene terpene before sexy time in the evening, when you are already tired, it may make you more sleepy and kill the vibe. While if your partner vaporises exactly the same strain but is wide awake and having trouble winding down and relaxing, it may add to their experience and help them get into the flow. It's just like any other sexual preference: some people are turned on by foot worship, whereas other people can't fathom what is so sexy about feet but maybe dirty talk or dressing up is their thing. The bottom line is: the best sex is what works best for you, whatever that may be.

My advice is that the best way to avoid a sex cannabis fail is to try the exact product and strain on your own first and see how it makes you feel. If you like the results, the next step would be to try it with your partner, as long as they are comfortable with the idea. Even if they do not want to try cannabis themselves, if it makes you feel good and they are supportive, then why not! Both parties do not necessarily have to partake, although some couples will say that they enjoy using cannabis together as a tool, and that it gets them on the same wavelength before sex. It's really a personal preference and there are no right or wrong decisions.

If you do try cannabis with a partner during sexy time and you experience a negative effect, often it is due to too much THC for you or the situation. This can result in feelings of paranoia and anxiety, as well as feeling very unsexy or turned off. The best thing to do in these scenarios is to express how you are feeling to your partner and take time out before proceeding. Never force it or keep going if something is not feeling right, just like any other sexual situation where something feels off. It's your body and your choice, always, and you get to change your mind if something suddenly stops feeling good! If this happens when you are self-pleasuring, again don't force things. Stop and relax; you can take some CBD to help counter the THC effects, practise deep relaxing breaths, put on some calming music or do whatever makes you feel good and grounded. If you have tried THC a few times for sex and it just didn't agree with you, stick to CBD products from hemp, which may still help enhance your feelings of relaxation and enjoyment without the THC effects.

There are no studies on the best sex strains as far as vaporised cannabis goes, but advice from cannabis sexuality coaches and self-reports, as well as what I tell my patients and clients, is all along the same lines: choose a strain based on how you want to feel during sexual play and what the typical barriers are for you (if any!) to getting in the mood. For example, if you are trying to get frisky in the evening and fatigue is a barrier, you may want to try a more sativa-dominant labelled strain with citrusy terpenes to give you a bit of a boost. If anxiety is a main factor, you may want to choose something more calming (with soothing terpenes like myrcene, linalool, or something labelled as an indica) to get out of your head and into exploring your body and your pleasure. The best thing is to choose a product and test it out in a small dose to see how it makes you feel. You can even keep a strain journal just for sex or for general cannabis uses and effects so you have a record of which strains you prefer for what.

Taking THC by mouth

Cannabis oils and sublingual tinctures tend to work a bit faster than capsules, so may be best for sex. In general, for sexual enhancement, if you are new to THC I advise you to start with a strain that contains both THC and CBD, to avoid THC overmedication (which can feel unsexy for some people). For example, start with a high-CBD oil or tincture (or one with a 1:1 CBD to THC ratio) and begin with a dose equal to 2 mg of THC. Take it 30–60 minutes before 'playtime' starts to allow it to start kicking in.

Vaporising THC

Choose a strain higher in CBD and lower in THC, such as a 2:1 CBD to THC ratio or a balanced strain (i.e.1:1), and start with a single inhalation after packing the vaporiser with a matchstick-head-sized amount. Wait for 5 minutes or so before taking a second dose, and after 2–3 doses spaced 5–10 minutes apart, check in with how you feel

There are no studies to guide dosing during sex, and your reaction will be very person-dependent, so take the 'start low, go slow' approach and use a diary to record your preferred strains and the dosages that seem to make you feel good and enhance your pleasure.

THC topicals

If you don't want to ingest cannabis or vaporise it, but are curious to see how the effects of a bit of THC may affect local sensation in the genitals, then trying a topical cannabis personal lubricant or oil may be the thing for you (though obviously only if you are in a jurisdiction where it is legal through a recreational non-prescription dispensary).

THC has very little penetration through normal skin from a topical. However, intimate application areas – the skin of the vulva in women or the scrotum in men, for example – are more permeable (porous), and topical THC on these areas may cause blood vessels to open up (vasodilation) through the release of a chemical called nitrous oxide, although this hasn't been proven yet in humans. So far, that effect has been seen using THC eye drops in cows,[10] but a similar reaction in the permeable genital mucosa areas in humans is a potential explanation for the 'warm and tingly', extra-sensitive pleasant sensation people report when they use THC topical products on the vulva. From personal accounts, it seems that these effects are more noticeable in women than men generally. Although again there are not yet any studies in this area, many sex coaches with experience using cannabis for enhancing the sexual experience recommend applying topical cannabis products at least 30 minutes before intimacy to allow them to work their magic.

A good indication of the strength of a health trend is how many companies have applied for patents in that area. For cannabis topicals for sex, the list of patents is growing by the day, and includes patents for topical aphrodisiac cannabinoid compounds,[11] as well as cannabis condoms[12] for enhancing pleasure and apparently helping with erectile dysfunction (again, we need more studies for definitive proof).

Because it may be possible for THC to enter the bloodstream from topical applications on mucous membranes and genital areas (athough still pretty unlikely in measureable amounts), if you are an athlete or likely to be drug tested for any reason, it may be safest to avoid any products with THC, even topically for sex.

Again, if you don't have access to legal THC-containing products, or can't use them, don't despair! There are many hemp-derived full-extract CBD products out there too that may also have local anti-inflammatory effects and make things feel nicer, even if it's just by virtue of being a good-quality non-irritating lubricant.

For additional information, see references[13, 14, 15, 16, 17, 18, 19, 20, 21, 22, 23].

CHAPTER FIFTEEN

BETTER GUT HEALTH

In most traditional medicine systems, including Chinese traditional medicine and Ayurveda, Indian herbal traditional medicine, the gut, or the gastrointestinal system, is the star of the show, and when a symptom arises is the first thing to treat. I studied Ayurvedic medicine in India, and my first integrative medicine mentor was also a doctor of Chinese medicine, so these ideas are something I was exposed to very early on in my medical career. Traditional ideas about gut health being relevant to overall health were still considered quite out there when I started practising mainstream medicine just over ten years ago. However, in the past few years, the mainstream research proof for this idea of gut health being directly related to overall health has finally caught up with what Indian and Chinese medicine doctors have known for over a thousand years.

I put a focus on gut health as a marker of overall health in treating my patients from the very beginning. I firmly believe that issues such as leaky gut and IBS are holistic health issues affecting both mental and physical health, and are not just confined to the intestines. Time and time again, when we started to repair a dysregulated gut in my practice, we found that symptoms were alleviated but also that the patient's mood and energy levels made a dramatic improvement. Even skin improved. This gut health protocol did not include any Western medicine drugs and was based on what I had learned from integrative medicine about treating the gut, doing things like repairing the lining, restoring healthier microbiome (the mix of gut bacteria inside our bodies) and removing irritants. We also used evidence-based mind-body approaches and lifestyle change to reduce the stress burden, which has a toxic effect on the gut just as it does on our brain and the rest of our body.

Years before I started prescribing cannabis, many of my patients were already using it to self-medicate their gut issues. They would confide in me how well it worked to control symptoms, especially when they were able to find, through trial and error, a strain that didn't make them feel high or give them the munchies (which was a major downside since it made them crave the bad carbs and inflammatory foods that they needed to avoid while healing their gut!). Back before medical cannabis was mainstream, this self-medication was a guessing game, since black market and home-grown cannabis was not tested for THC, CBD or terpene content (which still remains tricky to test for in big batches). When I started prescribing cannabis, we were able to target the type of product to the symptom, getting impressive results on gut symptoms where drugs had failed quite miserably on their, alongside the other natural approaches and often, in cases of severe gut diseases like inflammatory bowel, combining western medicine drugs with medical cannabis for better results and less side effects. I wasn't reinventing the wheel, since cannabis for gut issues is one of the oldest recorded uses. I was just rediscovering and honing it for the modern era.

The gut brain and gut–brain axis

Most people have had a 'gut feeling' about something, or experienced butterflies in their stomach when nervous or excited. It turns out that the gut actually has its own nervous system and our gut is pretty smart, with its own little brain, which scientists often call the 'second brain'. The gut brain and our actual brain have a two-way communication superhighway connecting them, called the gut–brain axis, and what affects one brain affects the other too. One of the first discoveries about this connection was that many of our brain chemicals, called neurotransmitters, are actually made *in* the gut, including over 80% of our happy hormone serotonin. And that's not all – the microbes in our gut are also a part of this gut–brain axis and can actually have a huge influence on not just physical health but also our mental health.[1] Scientists are starting to call some types of gut bacteria 'psychobiotics', meaning that they affect our psyche or mental health.

The ECS and gut health

The missing piece of the puzzle for gut–brain health was the discovery that the overarching regulatory system that appears to control the entire gut–brain axis and protect the gut is none other than our endocannabinoid system. The gut is packed full of cannabinoid receptors, which plant cannabinoids like CBD and THC interact with. The CB1 receptor seems to be particularly important in the anti-inflammatory effect seen with both CBD and THC in the gut,[2] but overall, the endocannabinoid system functions in the gastrointestinal (GI) system are wide-reaching in how they control everything from gut motility (how fast things like food move through the gut) to inflammation and pain.[3]

Medical cannabis as well as CBD products from hemp may have a major role to play in general gut health as well as actually treating specific disease of the gut. Due to the fact that until recently medical cannabis was not legal in most places, the research is still in its infancy, but studies are promising. If you are interested in learning more about them in detail, refer to the references for this chapter.[4, 5]

The current preliminary evidence in the published research supports the idea that cannabinoids can help in a variety of gut illnesses, including IBS, inflammatory bowel diseases such as Crohn's and ulcerative colitis, chronic nausea and chronic abdominal pain.[6] It can also help ease gut side effects of chemotherapy drugs in cancer treatment and help reduce the need for other pain drugs such as opioids, which often have severe gut side effects (e.g. constipation). I believe medical cannabis, while not a permanent cure (at least not that we can prove so far!), should be offered or at least discussed first, alongside other approaches, not last, in the treatment of gut disorders, due to its high safety and effectiveness when compared to the best drugs available.

Leaky gut

Leaky gut is an issue where the gut lining starts to become more permeable, or porous, allowing many things that shouldn't be able to leave the gut into the rest of the body. This is due to the loosening of something called the tight junctions,[7] which are like closely packed soldiers keeping everything (including invaders like bacteria, fungi and viruses) in the gut lumen where it belongs. The end result of these tight junctions getting lax is an inflamed, leaky gut lining in the small or large bowel (or both). The cycle of leakiness and inflammation is thought to be fuelled by proteins from certain foods, toxins, bacteria and other material such as inflammatory chemicals and growth factors from the bowel contents entering the rest of the body through the gut wall, gaining access to the blood and lymphatic system and causing immune reactions – setting the scene for a systemic chronic disease state that may manifest as anything from IBS to major depression, brain fog and chronic fatigue.[8, 9, 10, 11, 12, 13]

Until recently, the concept of leaky gut was marginalised by Western medicine, although integrative medicine and naturopathic physicians had been successfully treating patients with the issue for years for many seemingly unrelated symptoms. However, in the past ten years, it has been increasingly validated.

Related to leaky gut is an issue known as leaky brain. This is a theory gaining more evidence in which a leaky gut causes proteins, toxins and other inflammatory chemicals to gain entry into the brain via a similar filtration system that also becomes leaky. According to recent preliminary research by leading brain health researchers Dr Dale Bredesen and Dr David Perlmutter, leaky brain, if left untreated, may contribute to the development of brain problems ranging from depression to Alzheimer's. For this reason, they believe patients with unexplained neurological and mental health symptoms such as major depression should be tested and treated for leaky gut as well. The science of how this works is still in quite an early stage, but I have certainly seen some big shifts in patients over the years by incorporating a gut health approach for symptoms seemingly unrelated to the gut, especially in the mental health realm.[14]

If you think you may suffer from leaky gut, it is important to work with a health practitioner who understands this disorder and get on a gut health programme that includes diet and lifestyle change. You should also be checked for chronic gut infections or candida overgrowth, which may require an additional layer of the gut healing protocol.

Using cannabis for leaky gut

Cannabinoids may play a role in helping reduce leaky gut, inflammation and gut symptoms. I have found it to be an incredibly useful tool for my patients and clients who are going through a gut healing protocol. So far, there are no large published studies in humans, but *in vitro* studies have shown that both THC and CBD can reduce leaky gut or intestinal permeability from inflammation.[15] Generally I recommend a high-CBD oil or capsule taken 2–3 times a day to help with leaky gut. Vaporised cannabis can also be very helpful in relieving symptoms quickly, if needed for acute post-eating symptoms such as fatigue or bloating, and if available where you are by prescription.

Inflammatory bowel disease, including Crohn's

For centuries, the cannabis plant has reportedly been used medicinally for symptoms that would now be recognised as inflammatory bowel disease, or IBD. This is a term for a group of inflammatory autoimmune disorders of the gut, the most common forms being Crohn's and ulcerative colitis. IBD can involve severe diarrhoea, often with blood, abdominal pain, fatigue, weight loss and malnutrition, and can even in some cases cause life-threatening complications.

The cause of IBD is multifactorial, with a genetic and environmental component. Leaky gut (see above) is now thought to play a role in triggering it if there is already a genetic predisposition, leading to an abnormal immune response to foods and other proteins. Because of this, IBD is often termed an autoimmune disorder and can overlap or accompany other autoimmune diseases or psoriasis (see Chapters Sixteen and Seventeen if this is you). Many patients with IBD are already self-medicating with cannabis.[16]

In one study of treatment-resistant Crohn's where other drugs had failed, patients were given either THC cigarettes or a placebo.[17] The smoked THC led to a reduction in steroid use and improvements in sleep and symptoms, and no side effects were noted, but the study was only a short-term one so the long-term effects on those patients were not known.

Confusingly, in another study that looked at self-reported self-medication with black market cannabis in patients diagnosed with Crohn's, cannabis improved symptoms but was associated with a higher risk of needing surgery.[18] One of the reasons for this may be the type of cannabis and possible contaminants being used, as well as other factors that were not controlled for since it was an observational study using a survey, but it is hard to say for sure.

We know that in animal models, CBD can normalise motility (i.e. help with diarrhoea) and reduce inflammation.[19] In another animal study, a combination of THC and CBD was found to have an anti-inflammatory effect in mice with IBD (colitis).[20]

In humans, a recent placebo-controlled trial in ulcerative colitis concluded that a high dose of a CBD-rich medical cannabis capsule may be beneficial in treating ulcerative colitis symptoms, but that more studies are needed.

So far, we do not have published evidence that cannabis in any form can cure IBD or change the disease progression permanently.[21] However, I have found that adding a high dose of a high-CBD oil to treatment in some of my patients with treatment-resistant IBD means they have been able to be weaned off their steroids. High-CBD oil has also appeared to help normalise bowel function significantly (i.e. reduced pain and diarrhoea), which in itself is life-changing if you have severe IBD.

Alex's story

Alex came to see me because of his severe Crohn's disease. He was already on the best available drugs for Crohn's, known as biologics. Yet he still needed regular steroid pills every few months, which had quite horrible side effects of weight gain, problems with his blood sugar, sleep disruption and mood swings. However, there was nothing else that had really worked well to control the pain and diarrhoea, so he stayed on the drugs. He hadn't slept more than a few hours at a time for the past year, due to having to get up to use the toilet. He was exhausted and nutritionally deficient. He also needed to take opioid painkiller pills to help slow down the gut motility and ease his severe pain, and these were having side effects that he said made him feel 'like a zoned-out zombie'. He had used smoked cannabis recreationally on a regular basis when he was at university, and thought it might have been keeping his Crohn's symptoms under control, but he stopped smoking cannabis altogether after being told by his doctor that it was dangerous for his health and an addiction risk. He believes his disease got 'way worse' after that, although until we discussed the timeline in detail, he had never really thought about the coincidence between stopping smoking cannabis and his Crohn's flares worsening.

We decided to add medical cannabis using high-CBD, low-THC capsules three times a day at first, and a small dose of a high-THC oil before bedtime to help with his sleep disturbance and night pain. For the acute pain spasms, after adjusting to the cannabis oil, we also added a small amount of vaporised cannabis using a balanced strain (1:1 CBD to THC). I also added a high-dose curcumin supplement to the mix, which is a potent anti-inflammatory in the gut.

Within three months, Alex no longer needed the steroids, and after six months, he was sleeping through the night again. It was pretty life-changing, especially for his self-confidence and in his personal life with his partner. It also transformed his career, allowing him to work a normal day without running to the toilet every hour. This has previously caused him to have to leave his office job and work from home. Alex continues to use medical cannabis alongside his biologics (immune system modulating drugs) and anti-inflammatory suppositories (so far there have been no issues with combining them) and is still in remission almost three years later. Despite the occasional short-lived mild flare-up, he has had no need for steroids or adding new drugs to control his symptoms.

Using cannabis for IBD

For IBD, I generally recommend using a high-CBD oil or capsule by mouth as the mainstay of cannabis treatment, and then vaporised cannabis to break through the more acute symptoms of pain and to help increase appetite, using a balanced 1:1 strain. Some patients have reported a benefit from home-made high-dose-cannabis rectal suppositories, although no studies are yet published for this use. Generally speaking, high doses of cannabis with even significant THC seem to be able to be used rectally with less chance of impairment or intoxication than if taken orally. THC is generally less absorbed via this rectal route as far as we know, with more remaining in the gut, when compared with taking it by mouth.

IBS

IBS, or irritable bowel syndrome, is a functional gut disorder with symptoms ranging from food intolerance, gas and bloating to diarrhoea and constipation, abdominal pain and sometimes nausea. The worst thing about getting a diagnosis of IBS is that there are no solutions offered by Western medicine that are effective for most people and have a low side-effect profile. People are often told just to live with it. I have been treating IBS using an integrative medicine framework for almost a decade and have an entire IBS programme I put patients on. This includes many of the leaky gut methods as well as evidence-based mind-body approaches (gut-directed hypnotherapy), stress reduction and nutritional approaches. In addition, I have found that medical cannabis can alleviate symptoms as part of this more holistic approach. In many cases cannabis can replace the pharmaceutical drugs patients have been put on.

One of the reasons why cannabis works on these symptoms is that IBS may be a form of CEDS, or clinical endocannabinoid deficiency syndrome, a concept pioneered by Canadian medical doctor and cannabis medicine researcher Dr Ethan Russo and others.[22] Recent research has also found that cannabinoids can block gut pain signals,[23] and that a deficiency of cannabinoids (low cannabinoid tone) may contribute to chronic pain syndrome as well as problems with gut motility, which are both seen in irritable bowel syndrome. If this is the case, it may help explain why current drug approaches are usually ineffective, since we lack drugs that can rebalance endocannabinoid levels. Cannabis can work wonders almost immediately for some patients with IBS; even minutes after using it vaporised for the first time they can get some relief, something I also see in fibromyalgia and chronic migraine, which are the two other proposed CEDS disorders.[24]

Using cannabis for IBS

For IBS, I generally recommend using a high-CBD oil or capsule by mouth as the mainstay of treatment, and then vaporised cannabis for more acute symptoms of pain, using a balanced 1:1 strain.

Gastritis/GERD/heartburn

GERD, which stands for gastroesophageal reflux disease, and the more general term heartburn refer to a cluster of disorders involving food contents backing back up into the oesophagus from the stomach. This can happen due to an anatomical reason (called a hiatus hernia) or for other reasons related to diet or lifestyle. Symptoms can include:

- frequent heartburn, a burning feeling in your chest or throat
- a feeling of discomfort in the upper stomach like you are always full
- nausea
- regurgitating food or stomach contents
- sore throat
- difficulty swallowing (dysphagia)
- feeling like there's a lump in your throat
- damaged teeth from stomach acid
- chest pain that can mimic a heart attack in severe cases
- bad breath

Gastritis, which often has overlapping symptoms, is an inflammation of the stomach lining and can be due to a number of factors, including too much stomach acid, alcohol intake or an infection.

There are no big studies published yet on cannabis for the treatment of gastritis, GERD or heartburn. However, there is some research[25] to show that cannabis use decreases the risk[26] of alcohol-induced gastritis in alcoholics. I have treated many patients with medical cannabis for chronic pain conditions using a high-CBD cannabis oil. As a secondary benefit, I have had some patients report their GERD symptoms also improved, without any other changes to medication. I have also seen one case of severe gastritis where a patient tried a home-made cannabis oil and found it effective so came to me for help getting medical cannabis. We discussed the fact that there was no published literature to prove that it would help, but because he had tried everything else, we decided to give it a go. Over a three-month period, the cannabis oil reduced his symptoms more than anything else he had tried, with zero side effects. It may be that cannabis helps by reducing inflammation, since the gut lining in those with GERD and related symptoms has been shown to be impaired.[27]

In contrast to these positive effects, I have had one patient who started to experience GERD symptoms after starting a high-CBD cannabis oil for his chronic pain. A few colleagues have reported similar (but rare) cases in private communication, but these have not been published. The problem in each of these cases was solved by using oral capsules rather than an oil under the tongue or by mouth. The two explanations for this may be either a rare oral allergy to a cannabinoid or other plant chemical itself when coming in direct contact with the mucosa lining the mouth and upper oesophagus, or an oral allergy to the vehicle oil (coconut or flax oil being the two so far that may have been the issue). If available, a transdermal patch may be another good option to try instead.

Using cannabis for gastritis/GERD/heartburn

You can try starting with a high-CBD low THC medical cannabis oil or capsule (or a hemp CBD product for a non-prescription option) taken twice daily and monitoring whether this improves symptoms over a trial period of few months. If so, continue this approach.

Chronic nausea

Nausea is another symptom controlled in the brain through the endo-cannabinoid system receptors in specific nausea centres. It is one of the oldest traditional medicinal uses for cannabis. In one survey study of medical cannabis patients,[28] nausea was the fifth most common reason for use. The anti-nausea effect of cannabis is more down to THC than CBD, as THC binds to the CB1 receptors in these nausea centres. The easing of nausea is thought to be down to this brain effect, since cannabis can actually delay stomach emptying, which would generally be expected to make the symptom worse, especially in cases where the nausea is part of a GI issue called gastroparesis, where the digestion is too sluggish.[29, 30]

I have had patients with functional gut issues, including chronic nausea, use cannabis, usually vaporised, as needed for their nausea flare-ups; these patients preferred it to pharmaceutical drugs when other natural remedies like ginger root had failed.

Using cannabis for chronic nausea

Even though THC seems to be the main anti-nausea compound, if you take a daily oral high-THC, low-CBD cannabis product in any form, you will be at increased risk of side effects from unopposed THC (i.e. unmitigated by CBD), such as intoxication or impairment. This will be the case especially if you are unused to THC. For some people, high THC may be contraindicated, so please read the caveats and cautions in Chapter Six before choosing a product, especially if you have any mental health or heart conditions. That being said, a good way to start is with a very small dose of a balanced 1:1 or 1:2 THC to CBD ratio product, increasing the dose ever so slowly over a period of weeks. If your nausea is only occasional and comes on quickly, trying a vaporised cannabis flower with the same ratio may also help, again starting with a very low dose.

Chemotherapy-induced nausea and vomiting

As I write this chapter, one of my best friends, also an integrative medicine doctor and a brilliant psychiatrist, is undergoing chemo-therapy for stage 4 lymphoma cancer, which has come back after five years of remission. A day before she was due to arrive in London from LA to visit me, I received a phone call from her in the middle of the night with the worst news ever: the cancer was back. Thankfully, it was not in her brain like last time and it was ultra-responsive to chemotherapy. The worst part last time was the side effects of the super-strong chemotherapy she had to undergo for over two years directly into her brain and body via a spinal infusion. The nausea and pain were crippling. So she started trying a very small dose of medi-cal cannabis oil on the bad days, and it has so far helped her nausea and sleep, although she preferred the very low THC varieties as she was very sensitive to THC.

One of the things I often get asked via email, and sometimes from patients on their first visit, is whether cancer patients can stop (or not even start) conventional treatment and just take cannabis as their sole treatment instead. This is something I do not recommend, since we do not have enough evidence to say whether cannabis may be able to treat or cure cancer as the primary intervention. Cannabinoids are very promising future therapy targets, but we still need further study to demonstrate which cancers might respond to them, what dose and what type of cannabis product would be used, as well as what ratio of THC to CBD, and which other cannabinoids and terpe-nes might be effective against a specific tumour or cancer type, as well as to understand how they interact with immunotherapy.

Treating cancer is extremely complex, and every tumour is differ-ent: even two breast cancer tumours can have different cannabinoid receptors on them, making them respond differently to cannabis. I have known people who missed (or nearly missed until I convinced them not to) critical treatment windows in a curable cancer because they opted out of conventional therapy; often my job is to convince them to do the conventional therapy and then add cannabis to help with side effects. Cancer is super-scary, and I wish there was a proven sure-fire way of treating it successfully without needing chemo drugs or radiation, because these treatments have serious and often long-lasting side effects, but we're not there yet.

I have, however, read case reports (and actually know a few of these success stories personally!) of people who successfully treated their cancers with cannabis oils on their own, usually very high doses of a home-made oil. These patients experienced what Western medicine would deem a miraculous recovery; some had very advanced cancers that were resistant to chemotherapy. Nothing brings me more joy than hearing of these success stories, and my hope is that one day we can understand why cannabis has worked in these cases, and how to make it a reliable treatment for certain cancers, and tailor the treatment to the tumour using cannabinoid therapy.

In the meantime, using cannabis to help with the side effects of cancer treatment is a great start and can help people finish their chemo when otherwise they would have been too ill to continue (I've had a few cases like this). Chemotherapy-related nausea and vomiting is one of the uses for medical cannabis with the strongest evidence base in the published literature. Multiple extensive studies show the effectiveness of cannabis in these patients, especially when other anti-nausea drugs do not offer enough relief or have intolerable side effects. I have used medical cannabis successfully to treat chemo-related nausea in many of my patients, even those who had already tried the synthetic drug version of THC alone (nabilone) and had to stop due to side effects or it not working well for them. In addition to nausea and vomiting, cannabis can also help with cancer- and cancer-treatment-related pain, including chemotherapy-induced nerve pain.[31]

Using cannabis for chemotherapy-induced nausea and vomiting

Before starting any cannabis or CBD product if you are undergoing active cancer treatment, always consult you doctor first. Generally, I stick to low dose cannabis oils during therapy, higher CBD during the day, and a small dose of a higher THC oil before bed to help with worry, anxiety and sleep disruption.

If using inhaled vaporised cannabis for more acute nausea or severe vomiting, it is crucial to only use gamma-irradiated cannabis[32] that has had moulds and microorganisms such as bacteria removed without harming the CBD or THC content (although it can reduce terpenes). Since cancer patients are in an immune-compromised state (low immune system), inhaling any microbes from the cannabis flower is potentially quite dangerous. This is why home-grown and black market non-medical-grade-tested and irradiated cannabis is not recommended for use by people with cancer or any other low-immune-system conditions (HIV/AIDs, immunodeficiency diseases, etc.). Again, before starting anything always consult with your doctor first.

Cannabinoid hyperemesis syndrome

We cannot talk about gut issues and cannabis without addressing the one area where cannabis can harm rather than help. This is a relatively rare condition called cannabinoid hyperemesis syndrome (CHS), or in plain language cannabis vomiting syndrome. This usually happens after a period of chronic regular cannabis use, and the vomiting cycles and nausea can often go on for weeks before someone seeks medical attention. It affects men more commonly than women and the exact cause is not fully understood. This syndrome is normally only seen with high-THC recreational cannabis use, but in rare cases it can affect patients using medical cannabis. It is important to say that I have never seen a case of this in my medical practice using medical cannabis under controlled conditions, nor, to my knowledge, have my colleagues who do the same.

Normally the treatment for CHS is stopping cannabis completely in the long term. In the short term, taking hot baths helps,[33] as well as using capsaicin from hot peppers. Both hot baths/showers and the pepper extracts may work via a special receptor called TRPV1, which interacts with the ECS.[34] Other treatments include rehydration to prevent complications. Anti-nausea drugs are often not effective in treating the symptoms, and stopping cannabis is the only cure. If you are unsure whether you may have experienced this issue, stop any cannabis and consult with your doctor, as this is one of the few contraindications to medical cannabis. Although hemp-based CBD oil may be OK for some people who have experienced cannabinoid hyperemesis, there are unfortunately no published studies to guide us here.

How to use CBD wellness products (hemp CBD) for gut issues and gut health support

CBD on its own has been found to have a profound anti-inflammatory effect, so may be helpful in a number of gut conditions where inflammation is playing a role. Many people who cannot access medical cannabis have reported a benefit in symptoms ranging from leaky gut to IBS using a CBD hemp oil.

- Try a full-spectrum or broad-spectrum CBD oil.
- Look for the anti-inflammatory terpene called beta-caryophyllene – this terpene is also found in black pepper and has a woody/ spicy aroma.

Starting dose and titrating up

Starting doses for gut health and gut symptoms can vary from person to person, but in general, try starting with 5–10 mg of CBD twice or three times a day with meals for a total of 10–30 mg/day, which is still quite a low dose. I always advise the 'start low, go slow' approach. Gradually increase the dose every few days depending on your symptoms and preference, using a symptom tracker to test how you feel:

- What symptoms specifically do you want to track, and is each one improving?
- Are there other non-gut symptoms you want to work on, such as stress, anxiety, energy, etc.? (If yes see the relevant chapters.)
- Are symptoms related to eating (worse/better after food)?

You can slowly keep increasing the dose each week until symptoms improve or just stay at a lower dose as part of a more general gut-health routine. CBD tends to work best when used consistently over weeks/months, not as a one-off rescue remedy. If you reach 60 mg total per day, stay here for another 4–6 weeks before increasing again, which will avoid increasing the dose unnecessarily and saves money!

For inflammatory pain, higher doses may be needed, especially if you are not adding any THC from a prescription cannabis product and you have gut inflammation as a primary issue.

Remember: there is no specific perfect dose that works for everyone exactly the same. Each person's endocannabinoid system balance is unique, so self-titration is the name of the game with CBD.

How to use medical cannabis products for gut health

Using medical cannabis can be especially good if you have already tried hemp CBD and not noticed a huge change. Adding some THC can be very beneficial if nausea or more severe pain or gut spasms are issues for you. CBD can buffer the psychotropic effect (e.g. feeling high) and possible side effects of THC and also works in synergy with CBD on pain and inflammation. Only try this under the supervision of a doctor and, of course, if medical cannabis (containing THC) is legal where you live.

- Start with a high-CBD cannabis oil or capsule as your base. This is the best starting product, taken by mouth, especially if you are unused to THC.
- Choose a strain high in CBD and very low in THC, such as a CBD to THC ratio of 20:1.
- Look for products rich in beta-caryophyllene for anti-inflammatory action.
- Average starting dose: 5–10 mg of CBD 2–3 times a day with meals.
- Stay at this dose for a few days to a week or slowly increase the dose every few days depending on your pain response and preference. Track your symptoms to test how you feel.

- If the high-CBD, low-THC product has no effect after a few weeks, or symptoms like nausea get worse, change to a balanced oil or capsule (CBD to THC ratio of 1:1 or 2:1).
- Dosing for night-time pain and sleep disruption: it is not uncommon for some types of chronic gut pain or other symptoms to disturb sleep and proper rest. If sleep is an issue, refer to Chapter Eleven for how to try a night-time dose of a higher-THC calming indica-labelled myrcene-rich cannabis product.

How to use vaporising cannabis flowers for acute nausea or gut pain

- This is best used as a rescue medicine for nausea or acute pain spasms.
- Generally, it can be an add-on to a base of cannabis oil, not the primary mode of medicating on its own, to minimise THC side effects and avoid a roller coaster of THC levels.
- Try starting with high-CBD, low-THC flowers (especially if you are new to THC), because THC from vaporised cannabis hits the brain faster than oils by mouth. Once you are used to this, you can move on to a balanced strain, which may work better for pain, especially if accompanied by spasm of the gut, since THC is an anti-spasmodic.
- If nausea is the main issue, you can try a strain with more THC, known as a balanced strain (CBD to THC ratio of 1:1), since THC has a better effect on nausea.
- Start with a matchstick-head-sized amount, especially if it is a strain with more THC.
- See Chapter Five for detailed cannabis vaporising instructions.

CHAPTER SIXTEEN

WORKING WITH AUTOIMMUNE CONDITIONS

Autoimmune diseases are cases where the immune system misreads its own signals and the body starts to attack itself. In more scientific terms, an abnormal response to normal body proteins causes the body to attack healthy tissue and cells, such as the joints in cases of rheumatoid arthritis, or in the case of systemic lupus erythematosus (SLE), to attack joints as well as major organs such as the lungs, heart and kidneys and cause whole-body inflammation. For all autoimmune conditions there are both genetic and environmental factors, and this group of diseases remains one of the biggest treatment challenges in modern medicine. Since the discovery of oral steroid drugs, the survival rate of autoimmune conditions has improved dramatically. In SLE, for example, before the discovery of steroids, the one-year survival rate[1] was less than 50% (meaning over half of people died within the first year of being diagnosed with SLE), whereas now, with the best conventional treatment and use of steroids, the ten-year survival rate is over 90%! However, steroids and many of the newer drugs needed to control the autoimmune symptoms can cause significant and often disabling side effects. That is why the use of alternative or complementary therapies is very common in SLE[2] as well as other autoimmune disorders, as people look for a less toxic option or at least as an add-on to pharma drugs.

Enter cannabis to the rescue once again, because in addition to potent anti-inflammatory properties, many cannabinoids also have immunosuppresive powers too. That may sound like a bad thing, but in autoimmune disorders, the immune system has become overactive and we are trying to calm it back down. That is what steroids and other drugs to treat these conditions do too, but at a huge side-effect cost to both brain and body. Oral steroids, for example, used chronically, can cause diabetes, prevent people from sleeping properly, and lead to depression and mood issues, weight gain and belly fat that refuses to budge despite diet and exercise.

The body's immune cells have both CB1 and CB2 receptors, and CB2 receptors[3] in particular seem to maintain balance and regulate healthy immune function. So we know the endocannabinoid system plays an important role in autoimmune disorders when this balance goes wrong. Using plant cannabinoids to help regain balance is less well understood in terms of published research, but I have found that they can be of enormous benefit in treating my patients with autoimmune disorders. They seem to work on the endocannabinoid system immune pathways as well as via other non-cannabinoid immune pathways that control things like chronic inflammation, which is a big issue in autoimmune diseases. We are still learning all the ways cannabis works on the immune system and don't have all the answers quite yet, but we do know that cannabinoids can affect various immune cells that can go wrong in immune dysfunction conditions, including T cells,[4] mast cells, immune cell chemicals including one called TNF alpha, and many others.

The preliminary evidence for cannabis medicines in autoimmune disease treatment is promising, but the amount of published data is still sparse, and much of it is pre-clinical, meaning done in a lab setting, or in animal models. This lack of big-study published evidence is due to the same common factors seen in other areas of cannabis medicine, i.e. cannabis being illegal and unable to be studied until very recently; and the fact that as a botanical medicine with hundreds of active compounds, it's difficult to study as easily as a single-ingredient drug. Rheumatologists (joint doctors) and other conventional medicine specialists who treat autoimmune diseases are often quoted as saying that cannabis has 'significant side effects'. That is then used as a reason why they don't recommend it, and they often even discourage their patients from trying it. I always find this quite interesting (as well as frustrating!), considering that most of the 'gold standard' therapy drugs they are using have significant risk of multiple serious side effects and can even include multi-organ toxicity. Cannabis has none of these toxicities to organs. This fear of cannabis in rheumatology, as in other specialities in medicine, comes in large part from a lack of understanding. This is starting to be acknowledged at last, and doctors are recommending more education for physicians around the endocannabinoid system[5] as well as in cannabis uses for autoimmune disease treatment, and some rheumatologists have started to consider cannabinoid therapy for their patients.

Ben's story

Ben was a patient I met through a cannabis advocacy group in the UK who had suffered from a form of SLE since he was 10 years old. When originally diagnosed, he diligently took the conventional medicine therapies for years, despite them unfortunately causing kidney damage, severe nausea and vomiting, weight loss and a variety of other serious symptoms. Eventually he found cannabis through a patient support group for his condition and began taking cannabis suppositories each day as well as vaporised cannabis for his pain, inflammation and disease, which affected his joints as well as various organs. After taking cannabis, he was able to function and eat, and although not quite pain free, he resumed a normal life. He could see friends and actually leave his house, which had become like a prison over the past five years.

Cannabis was like a miracle for him and his family, and yet his doctors still refused to acknowledge the difference it had made, which is how he became an advocate for medical cannabis and started to share his experience with other patients and doctors with an interest in cannabis medicine. His story is not rare. In my own practice in Canada, I have prescribed cannabis to many patients with autoimmune disorders including SLE, with incredible results, often shocking the other specialists involved in their care with their progress and ability to taper down many medications that were causing multiple side effects. The published research hasn't caught up with my clinical experience yet, but I have no doubt we will see this happen in the next few years.

Rheumatoid arthritis

Black market illicit use of cannabis for rheumatoid arthritis (RA) is widespread, and of those who use it for self-medication, 100% indicated that they found it made them either 'much better' (72%) or 'a little better' (28%) according to a recent poll.[6] Cannabis can help joint inflammation and pain via working with both CB1 and CB2 cannabinoid receptors in the joints,[7] and systemic anti-inflammatory effects have been seen with CBD. One study using Sativex,[8] which is a pharma cannabis medicine with a 1:1 ratio of THC:CBD, showed that it was effective at reducing both pain and actual disease activity and progression, and is well tolerated in RA. That is pretty great news considering the other top conventional drugs to treat RA and reduce disease activity have serious side-effect potential, ranging from severe drug reactions to organ toxicities and extreme fatigue. Another study looked at cannabinoid receptors in the joint fluid[9] and, based on its findings, predicted that for both RA and osteoarthritis, these cannabinoid receptors are a promising therapeutic target for treating joint pain and inflammation.

CBD has been shown to be effective against inflammatory arthritis in mice due to its immunosuppressive and anti-inflammatory effects,[10] and multiple animal studies show potential.

Rachel's story

Rachel was in her mid-twenties, and in many ways she was like any other 20 something: she loved music and hanging out with her friends, and was studying at university. However, unlike most of her peers, she had had to drop out of university twice due to her severe rheumatoid arthritis. She experienced crippling pain and fatigue that kept on progressing despite the maximum medical therapy she was on, including steroids nearly daily for the better part of the past few years, and biologics via intravenous infusion. She was severely disabled by her illness and, despite her good grades and natural academic aptitude, she could not finish her degree. She dreamed of being able to become a biologist and just be normal – practise yoga, go for a jog and join her friends at concerts. She had tried smoking cannabis only once, and didn't like the way it made her feel, so she never tried it again.

We discussed putting her on medical cannabis, and despite her initial hesitance because of her negative experience, she had an amazing response. In three months, she was off the steroids, and after six months, she felt normal for the first time in years. She rejoined her university degree course and could function nearly pain-free most days.

We used a high-CBD, low-THC oil and capsule regimen, and Rachel used inhaled cannabis with a bit more THC when she had bad pain and fatigue days. Just being able to stop the steroids made a huge difference to her sleep and mood – she no longer felt exhausted every morning, and her mild depression symptoms went away too. She continues to use cannabis alongside her biologics (immune system modulating drugs) with so far no issue, and feels that cannabis gave her her twenties back.

How to use CBD wellness products (hemp CBD) for inflammation

Hemp CBD wellness products are not meant to be a main treatment for a serious medical illness on their own. That being said, I have come across cases where people have used an over-the-counter high-quality, higher-dose hemp-based CBD product and found that it did decrease both pain and inflammation. This has often allowed them to stop other prescription pain pills and continue using CBD alongside other conventional medicine with fewer side effects than before they added it on.

- Try a full-spectrum or broad-spectrum CBD oil.
- Look for anti-inflammatory terpenes:
    - beta-caryophyllene – also found in black pepper; has a woody/spicy aroma

- myrcene – smells earthy/peppery, like hops, and is sedating, so good for night-time pain (may be too sedating for daytime); also has anti-inflammatory effect.

Starting dose and titrating up

Try starting with 10 mg of CBD first thing in the morning, at midday/early afternoon (12–2 p.m.) and at dinner time for a total of 30 mg/day. Especially if you are on other drugs for autoimmune disease, especially biologics, or are on drugs for blood clotting, always consult your doctor first and see Chapter Six for cautions.

Slowly increase the dose every few days. You may notice after 1–2 weeks that there is less inflammation and/or pain. You can slowly keep increasing the dose each week until symptoms improve.

Remember: there is no specific perfect dose that works for everyone exactly the same. Each person's endocannabinoid system and immune system balance is unique, and so far no studies have been published on the best doses for CBD in autoimmune diseases, so self-titration is the name of the game. As always, consult with your doctor before trying any new supplement or medication, since this is merely a guide and not medical advice

For maintenance: non-cannabis helpers to add

If pain or sleep are also issues, see the relevant chapters for details and tips.

- Anti-inflammatory herbs: turmeric whole-root tincture, high-dose curcumin, boswellia and bromelain.
- Get your vitamin D level tested. Keeping serum (blood) vitamin D levels around the 60–75 percentile (your doctor should know what this means and how to do it with you!) may improve pain scores in some people with inflammatory arthritis and autoimmune disease. Achieving this with vitamin D3 drops in oil form is the best way to ensure absorption, since the tablets are not well absorbed.

- Dietary modification for autoimmune disease: many people find that an elimination diet has some effect (in many cases a huge effect) on their symptoms and flare-ups. I recommend a trial of a quite strict diet that is a form of paleo eating (no grains or legumes or other specific foods that may trigger an autoimmune response), known as the AIP diet. When adhered to for a period of three months, this diet has been proven to decrease inflammation[11] in autoimmune diseases including Crohn's disease[12] and autoimmune thyroid disease, though I'm the first to admit it is very hard to stick to completely in the long run. You may find that by sticking to it 80% it may make a difference for you too; it's something to experiment with to find your best balance point.
- Adding in a high-potency omega-3 oil from krill (1g/day) has some positive effect in small studies with rheumatoid arthritis patients and is very safe, as well as being good for general brain wellness.

How to use medical cannabis products for autoimmune conditions

This is especially good if you have already tried hemp CBD and not noticed a huge change. Adding some THC can be hugely beneficial, and appears to works in synergy with CBD on autoimmune response, inflammation and pain. Only try this under the supervision of a doctor and, of course, if medical cannabis (containing THC) is legal where you live.

- Start with a high-CBD cannabis oil as your base for daytime pain. This is the best starting product, taken by mouth.
- Choose a strain high in CBD and very low in THC, such as a CBD to THC ratio of 20:1.
- Look for products rich in beta-caryophyllene for anti-inflammatory action, and other good daytime terpenes (see Chapter Five). CBG is also a potent anti-inflammatory, so look for strains rich in this cannabinoid too if possible.

- Average starting dose: 5–10 mg 3x/day with meals, so with breakfast, lunch and dinner.

Adding a THCA oil to the CBD base

THCA is the precursor to THC (see Chapter Three for a refresher) that was initially overlooked due to the fact that it was non-intoxicating. However, although there are no published studies yet for its use in humans, I have discovered clinically that adding a THCA oil to a high-CBD oil during the day often seems to help with autoimmune disease symptoms better than CBD alone in difficult-to-treat cases. Lab studies have shown that THCA is likely an immunomodulator, meaning it regulates the immune response, in addition to its known anti-inflammatory and anti-seizure effects.

I use the 'start low, go slow' approach when adding THCA, starting with between 2 and 4 mg 3x/day taken with the high-CBD oil. THCA oil (or capsules, where available) is often hard to find, but more medical cannabis suppliers are making it, especially in North America, and it has started to be added to the available medical cannabis prescription products in the UK too. It must be stored carefully to minimise degradation of the THCA into active THC.

Dosing for night-time pain and sleep disruption

It is very common for those suffering with autoimmune diseases to be affected by night pain and sleep disturbance, which may have a negative effect on inflammation and immune system function. That is why I always treat night pain and sleep from the get-go, with a night-time cannabis medicine dose using higher THC (unless there is a contraindication: see Chapter Six).

- Start with a balanced strain (i.e. a CBD to THC ratio of 1:1) or a high-THC, low-CBD cannabis oil.
- Look for calming terpenes like myrcene and linalool. CBN, which is low in raw cannabis but higher in older cannabis flower and oils as a breakdown product of THC, may enhance the sedative and pain-relieving qualities of the other cannabinoids.

- Start with 2 mg of THC and take one hour before bedtime.
- Stay at this dose for a few days to a week or slowly increase the dose every few days depending on your response and preference. Because there is also a small amount of THC in these oils, slowly titrate the dose up by a few mg each week, as everyone is slightly different in how they respond.

How to use vaporising cannabis flowers for inflammation and pain

This is the best mode of delivery for stopping acute inflammatory pain attacks that may come on suddenly. It should be an add-on to a base of cannabis oil, not the primary mode of use, to minimise side effects and avoid a roller coaster of THC levels.

- Start with high-CBD, low-THC flowers, especially if you are new to THC, because THC from vaporised cannabis hits the brain faster than oils by mouth.
- If this has no effect, you can try a strain with more THC, known as a balanced strain, with equal amounts of CBD and THC (i.e. 1:1).
- Start with a matchstick-head-sized amount, especially if it is a strain with more THC. Look for strains high in beta-caryophyllene, for anti-inflammatory effect.
- See Chapter Five for detailed cannabis vaporising instructions.

Topicals for joints

Topical products can be helpful for localised areas of joint swelling, inflammation and pain, especially in small close-to-the-surface joints like knees, wrists and hands, as well as ankles and feet. Muscle balms with CBD and menthol may also be helpful for the aches and pains that many people with autoimmune disease experience. These are extremely safe and can be applied to painful areas of muscle at any time, but may work best after a hot shower, when pores are open, although no studies have been done to confirm this. Using a topical that contains menthol and linalool may help the CBD penetrate slightly better into the skin. CBD has more penetrability than THC when used topically, but topical THC may also help inflammation (where legally available). Multiple animal studies have found that topical CBD preparations reduce joint swelling.

CHAPTER SEVENTEEN

SKIN CONDITIONS AND CBD

Our skin is the largest organ in our body, and it's also the first thing we show to the world. Everyone knows that when the condition of our skin is poor, it affects our confidence and sense of self. My first published research paper was about skin – specifically skin cancer and tanning parlour use – so it's an area of medicine I'm quite passionate about. Because I'm a medical doctor, I'm more concerned about skin health than about beauty, but let's face it, everyone wants to have better skin (or to keep skin looking amazing if you've already been blessed with a great complexion). The cool thing I have discovered about skin health, and what I like to think of as skin wellness, is that our skin is often a barometer for what is going on inside our bodies. When skin is healthy, it's also more luminous, less spotty and more youthful-looking, so health and beauty really do go hand in hand. I know that when I get run down, or am shifting through time zones doing lots of air travel and eating less than optimally, my skin and my digestion are the first things to get disrupted. My skin loses its glow, starts to look dull and tired, and my digestion gets sluggish. It's a sign for me to clean up my act!

And lo and behold – it turns out that we have cannabinoid receptors in all of the different complex cells that make up our skin.[1] We are just beginning to understand the myriad factors that control skin homeostasis, which keeps the skin's ecosystem in harmony. The endocannabinoid system of our skin is emerging as a key player in this balance: controlling normal skin barrier function, growth and maturation of different types of skin cells, and skin inflammation.

Because of their proven anti-inflammatory effects, topical cannabis products may be helpful for a number of skin conditions, such as
dermatitis and eczema (dry skin), psoriasis (possibly due to effects
on the skin's immune system), acne, excessive hair growth and even
some skin pre-cancers or early non-melanoma cancers. This is due
to the fact that all of these disorders share a dysregulation in the
skin's endocannabinoid system[1] or, as one researcher group calls it,
the cutaneous cannabinoid or cutannabinoid system for short.

The exact cannabinoid ratio and profile that would work best for
each of these conditions, or the optimal dose, is not yet known. There
are not yet any published studies on exact product and dosage in
humans with these skin issues. However, as a general rule, as with
any skin or topical application, choosing a high-quality product with
higher amounts of active ingredients – in this case including CBD
(and/or THC depending if it is legal without prescription where you
live) as well as other minor cannabinoids – along with a formulation
designed to enhance absorption is likely to produce greater effects.
Some very low-dose products where there is minimal CBD or other
cannabinoid content may not do much at all. In addition to the cannabinoid content, some products (often cheap ones, but not always)
may contain other common skin irritants or allergens.[2] These can also
affect skin barrier function and inflammation, so as with any skin product, quality is key.

In my medical practice in Canada, medical cannabis is usually for
ingestion, taken sublingually or vaporising at the time of writing. But
some of my patients have made their own topical balms from cannabis flower with good results on conditions such as psoriasis, eczema
and skin irritation. I have also used it myself topically (CBD oil) for
mild acne and thought it made some difference with no skin side
effects. That is what you call an 'N of one' study – i.e. one person
trying something and reporting that it worked. It is not very scientific,
but it is a start into inviting more research and interest into an area.
Many drug discoveries in medicine have started as an 'N of one'. In
the UK, I hear from many people, and have met many cannabis medicine advocates, who similarly use their own self-made home-grown

cannabis products successfully for skin conditions. In addition, people are using hemp-based CBD wellness products on their skin with very promising results based on their reports. Often people report that these products have helped when even prescription topical drugs had failed or caused skin side effects. We need more research into these applications to discover what may work best at which dose.

Topical CBD or THC, or both?

CBD, THC and other minor cannabinoids and certain terpenes may all have beneficial effects on the skin. Topical CBD and THC have both been shown to reduce skin inflammation,[3] and THC topically can be helpful for extreme itchiness (known to doctors as pruritus).

One study[4] showed that in addition to their better-known cousins, the minor cannabinoids CBG and CBGV may have potential in the treatment of dry-skin syndrome, whereas CBC, CBDV and especially THCV show promise to become highly efficient new anti-acne agents.

CBD has anti-acne and anti-inflammatory properties in preliminary research, which may be useful for all of the skin conditions below. This is why it is the hottest new ingredient in skincare products for both face and body. It is backed by published (although very preliminary) evidence of its biological activity in the skin. One study that used a CBD ointment in patients with either psoriasis, eczema or scarring[5] concluded that it significantly improved skin parameters and symptoms with zero side effects or toxicities. It's a great step forward for topical skin disorder treatment options, because many other strong topicals for acne, psoriasis and even eczema are very drying, considered possibly unsafe for pregnancy or may lead to thinning of the skin when used on a regular basis.

Acne

Acne is an inflammatory disease,[6] and CBD is a powerful anti-inflammatory plant chemical, both topically and ingested. Again, preliminary research suggests that it can help acne when applied topically, and it is a very safe treatment option when used along with other topical acne creams. The optimal dose is unknown, but choosing a higher-potency, high-quality product is a good starting point for finding the best option for you.

After forgoing hormonal methods to control my mild acne, I used a topical high-CBD cannabis product on my skin, combining it myself (DIY compounding, I like to call it!) before there was anything commercially available. When I ran out of it, or when I was in Bali where I couldn't take it, my mild acne would return and I would have to go back to a prescription topical. Sometimes, when I had access to both, I would even combine the prescription topical and the CBD DIY topical. One of the things I noticed personally with the CBD was that it didn't dry out or inflame my skin the way some of the prescription topical acne creams did. I'm a huge believer in its potential and have had many patients and clients who have had similar experiences. Now there are many commercially prepared cannabis and hemp-derived CBD skin products for acne better formulated for facial skin so you don't have to concoct your own!

For additional information, see references[7, 8, 9, 10].

Psoriasis

Psoriasis is a chronic inflammatory disease where the skin loses control over how fast the upper skin cells, called keratinocytes, turn over. This causes a build-up of this upper skin layer, resulting in psoriasis plaques, which are red or pink and scaling. The disease has a genetic as well as an environmental component. There is no cure, but I have seen cases of complete remission of the skin symptoms with an integrative medicine approach (not only cannabis), with patients often being able to dramatically reduce and minimise steroid creams and other drugs.

Treating psoriasis with pharmaceutical topicals and systemic medications often carries a high risk of toxicities and side effects, so any natural effective treatment is a welcome addition to a patient's regime. My patients with psoriasis suffer not just with the flaking, scaling plaques that in themselves cause itching and often painful irritation, but also with the secondary effects: having to deal with the reactions of others. Often people who don't know what psoriasis is see someone with the skin lesions and avoid them, fearing it is something contagious or infectious. This is of course not the case, but there is still a lot of social stigma around this disease and resulting social isolation. I have patients who refuse to go for a massage or even wear a sleeveless shirt in the hot summer months because they are embarrassed about their skin and the negative attention they have received in the past. These secondary social effects have a serious impact on mental well-being and self-confidence, as with all skin disorders, so I take treating them the best way possible very seriously.

Along with cannabis, which can be a great help, I also take a more holistic integrative/functional medicine approach and address stress factors, as well as looking into the possibility of leaky gut playing a role, due to the microbiome effect (see Chapter Fifteen). This is a reason why seeing a health practitioner or integrative/functional medicine doctor for a full assessment and plan can be so helpful in psoriasis and similar chronic skin disorders in addition to the normal Western medicine tools.

Again, the exact dose and product that works best for psoriasis is not yet known. However, you can try starting by softening the plaques and then applying a product that is made for enhanced skin absorption, using a generous amount twice a day all over the affected areas. This is likely the best way to see a significant change. So far, studies have mostly focused on CBD, but other cannabinoids, including THCA, have been shown to be able to inhibit a chemical that is involved in many inflammatory disorders, including psoriasis.[11] It has anti-psoriasis properties too, such as inhibiting an inflammatory chemical called TNF alpha.

Some of my patients in Canada who take oral medical cannabis for chronic pain have psoriasis too. They would often show me the before and after photos of their skin flare-ups, and it was noticeable that their skin cleared up considerably after starting medical cannabis for their chronic pain, including high-CBD products. So combining topical CBD plus an oral medical cannabis oil or hemp CBD oil daily may give the best results, though there are no studies yet, just clinical experience. You can try starting at 15–30 mg/day by mouth and increase the dose based on your response over a period of weeks and months, looking for an effect after three and then six months of daily use.

For additional information, see references[12, 13, 14, 15, 16].

Eczema

Eczema is another inflammatory skin condition where the skin becomes very dry, dehydrated and inflamed, impairing the normal barrier function and in extreme cases resulting in painful, cracked and even bleeding skin and recurrent skin infections, as well as extreme itchiness or pruritus that often requires potent anti-itch drugs. Recent research[17] supports the idea that the endocannabinoid system plays a role in eczema, which suggests that the use of cannabis may be helpful. Preliminary research has shown that topical CBD as well as topical THC have anti-eczema effects in mice and in cells, but human studies beyond case reports are still lacking.[18,19]

As with psoriasis, the exact product and dosage is not yet reported in a research study. You can start by choosing a high-quality product; using a generous amount twice daily all over the affected areas is likely the best way to get a significant result. Taking oral CBD from hemp or a high-CBD medical cannabis oil may help reduce flares due to stress and anxiety, one of the most common triggers for eczema (for dosing for stress and anxiety, please refer to Chapters Eight and Nine).

Skin wounds and other skin diseases

Pain and delayed healing in topical skin wounds from a variety of conditions is a difficult issue to treat. However, topical cannabinoid creams may play a role in reducing pain[20] and speeding up healing time[21] in pyoderma gangrenosum (a rare skin condition with large painful sores) and various skin-blistering diseases (where the skin develops painful fluid-filled blisters or sacs that can cause scarring), with the added benefit of reduced opioid painkiller usage in these painful skin disorders.

Skin cancers and pre-cancers

The published research on the ability of cannabis topicals to treat or even cure skin cancers is only very preliminary, but thousands of case reports with photographic anecdotal evidence are hard to ignore. In mice, it has been found that cannabinoid drugs used topically have anti-skin-tumour activity.[22] Although it is too early to recommend topical cannabis products as a primary treatment for skin cancers of any type, it is possible that using a topical cannabis skin cream over the years may help with preventing sun- and UV-related pre-cancerous non-melanoma skin lesions (actinic keratoses, or AKs as they are known for short) from turning into cancer. It's still not proven in the published literature, but doctors (including myself) who treat people with medical cannabis all have stories from patients who used a topical cannabis product on their own to treat AKs. They report that they were able to get rid of the lesions completely with repeated applications over a number of weeks and needed no further treatment. It should be noted that these AK lesions are very different from invasive, deep or more serious skin cancers, which would likely not respond to a purely topical treatment this way.

How to use cannabis for skin conditions

- Choose a topical product suitable for the condition you wish to treat. For example, if you are trying to target acne, choose a high-quality tested product for acne-prone skin and look for other synergistic ingredients such as salicyclic acid, niacinamide or probiotics. If you are trying to treat large areas of the body for eczema, dry skin or psoriasis, choose a product made for the body and formulated for enhanced absorption if possible.

- Apply liberally multiple times a day.
- For psoriasis, a CBD body lotion may be tried in combination with prescription topicals such as vitamin D analogues to possibly improve the effect (although no studies on this yet) but always consult your doctor first.
- To help with stress-induced flare-ups of eczema, psoriasis or other stress-related skin issues, consider following the guidelines in Chapters Eight and Nine for using an oral CBD oil from hemp or high-CBD medical cannabis oil by prescription (if available).

Ingredients to avoid in your skincare regimen

Just because a product has CBD in it doesn't mean it's safe or effective! I have seen many products on shelves claiming to help with skin irritation that also contained multiple skin irritants and other potentially unhealthy chemicals, so read the label on the product you choose just as carefully you would with your food. All the following products can potentially cause skin irritation in some users, so they are best avoided, especially if your skin is particularly sensitive.

- parabens
- imidazolidinyl urea
- quaternium-15
- formaldehyde
- 'fragrance mix'

CHAPTER EIGHTEEN

HELP FOR EPILEPSY AND SEIZURES

If there is one use for cannabis and CBD that seems to grab the headlines again and again, it is the ability of the drug to ease seizures in treatment-resistant epileptics. Epilepsy is actually a broad group of brain conditions involving seizures of many different types and causes. Regardless of the exact type and cause, medical cannabis and particularly high-CBD cannabis can help reduce seizures, often dramatically, and even when modern drug cocktails are failing. This is something I have seen again and again first-hand with my patients in Canada, and then again in the UK advising on treatment-resistant epilepsy cases and the use of medical cannabis in certain forms of childhood epilepsy.

In many cases of childhood epilepsy, the children have been close to death, or in and out of intensive care weekly. They were on enormous doses of drugs and steroids, causing side effects ranging from mood changes and even psychotic episodes to impact on growth and development. They have gone from having no hope of a normal childhood to getting seizure control for the first time in years by adding high-CBD medicinal cannabis oil. It has also in many cases allowed them to come off all the steroids and many of the other drugs while keeping the seizures to a minimum. Taking cannabis has allowed them to return to school and a normal life.

For these patients and their families, it feels like a miracle and is often the end of a parent's worst nightmare. But many thousands of children still cannot get access to this life-changing treatment; in fact that is the case for most, despite the growing body of evidence.

The ECS and epilepsy

So how does cannabis actually work for epilepsy? It all comes back to our endocannabinoid system, which helps balance our brain and body, including healthy seizure-free brain communication and function. Seizures are the result of a burst of abnormal electrical activity that can start in one part of the brain and then spread. This burst of activity is due to overexcitability of brain cells, essentially an overcommunication issue, something that is controlled by the endocannabinoid system. In essence, it seems that a healthy endocannabinoid system acts as a circuit breaker,[1] preventing the abnormal bursts of electrical overactivity that cause the seizures.

Seizure symptoms can vary widely depending on what part of the brain is affected. Symptoms of generalised seizures include full-body muscle spasms, body stiffness and loss of consciousness. Other forms of seizures that are more focused in the brain may just look like the person is daydreaming or zoned out. Whatever the cause and type of seizure, the endocannabinoid system plays a critical role in this process,[2] according to an ever-growing and compelling body of research. For example in animal studies, blocking CB1 cannabinoid receptors[3] in the brain resulted in severe seizures, meaning that the functioning of the CB1 receptors and the cannabinoids is critical to normal seizure-free brain activity. Other studies in humans so far have discovered reduced endocannabinoid functioning in the brain[4] and spinal fluid[5] of those with certain types of epilepsy, suggesting that an endocannabinoid deficiency may be involved.

The evidence for CBD in seizures

We reached a very important turning point in 2017 regarding the efficacy of CBD in particular on reducing seizures, with three high-quality 'best-evidence' type of studies (randomised placebo-controlled trials)[6] on a pharma drug made from plant-derived CBD called Epidiolex, a product used in patients with specific seizure disorders called Dravet syndrome and Lennox-Gastaut syndrome. In these studies the high-dose CBD was found to be effective in reducing seizures against a placebo arm, or sugar pill. This now gives us the beginnings of what is known, even in the most conservative mainstream medical circles, as level 1 evidence that CBD works for seizures.

The way cannabinoids, and CBD in particular, actually stop the abnormal firing and overcommunication issue in the brain cells is not yet fully understood on a micro level. However, the current research[7] points to many different brain effects from cannabinoids, including neuroprotective effects, anti-inflammatory pathways, and effects on many other proteins and even serotonin (happy hormone) pathways.

Julie's story

The first time I saw Julie with her mother (who was also her caregiver), she didn't really communicate verbally. Her mother did most of the talking. Julie was 25 years old and unable to live independently due to her severe epilepsy, for which she took a strong cocktail of drugs, without great success in reducing the seizure frequency dramatically and also with many side effects. Her mother said that the drugs made her 'like a zombie' and unable to care for herself, and they had not stopped her daily seizures. Life was a struggle for them both, as she'd had to quit her job to care for Julie, and money was now very tight, another pressure on top of everything else. Julie loved dogs, and her mother knew she would benefit from an assistance dog, but she was too unwell to qualify for the programme and was told it was unlikely to happen in the future. They had heard about medical cannabis for seizures and wanted to try it, and their neurologist had agreed and referred her to the clinic. We decided to start with a very high-CBD, low-THC cannabis oil, and worked with her other doctors as we added it, to make sure her seizure medication was still in the safe range.

Over the course of the next year, Julie's seizures became much better controlled, until they were down to one seizure only every three to four months and she no longer required dramatic medical intervention to stop them. She reduced the doses of many of her other medications slowly under medical supervision as she increased the cannabis oil, and a year after starting medical cannabis treatment she was a changed woman. She could speak to me normally, had become more independent and was considering moving out of her mother's house with some part time assistance. She had qualified for an assistance dog and was even looking at getting a part-time job. These were things she'd never thought would be possible. She no longer seemed depressed and was able to start having more outings in the community and more social interactions. For both Julie and her mother, the change felt like a miracle, as it had given both of them their life back. Her epilepsy would never be cured, but cannabis kept it at bay and had radically transformed her quality of life – and she experienced zero side effects from it, which for an epilepsy treatment was pretty much unheard of.

Alfie's story: the fight for cannabis medicine for kids in the UK

When I moved to the UK and started getting involved in medical cannabis training for doctors and in cannabis education, I met many incredible families and children living with drug-resistant forms of epilepsy where medical cannabis had been the only thing that helped. One of these children was Alfie Dingley. His mum, Hannah Deacon, had campaigned tirelessly to fight for the rights of children with this condition to access medical cannabis as a last-resort treatment. Her fight, and those of other parents of children with seizure disorders where cannabis has been hugely beneficial but were denied the therapy, had a huge role in the British government changing the law around cannabis to make medical cannabis legal in the UK in November 2018.

I started working with Alfie's doctors, helping them to find the best cannabis dosages and products to control and minimise his seizures. That was often tricky due to being able to access only a limited number of products. Alfie responded incredibly well to medical cannabis, which dramatically reduced his seizures when other drugs had failed, and with few side effects. This was after he had been having hundreds of seizures each week, and had been in and out of intensive care, unable to attend school, as well as suffering severe mental and physical side effects from steroids and drugs that just were not working for his type of epilepsy.

It has been a privilege to be able to help Alfie and the many other children like him across the UK who need better access to medical cannabis. Public and doctor education, working with government policy groups and supporting research are all helping, but we still have a long way to go until all these children have the medicine they need.

Another family I met was able to get a medical cannabis prescription for their very sick son, but the cost was so expensive (around £2000 per month on average) that they had to remortgage their house to pay for it. The problem still remains that most epilepsy doctors are afraid of medical cannabis, especially when used in children, because they have a poor understanding of how cannabis works and were not taught anything about it in medical school. To make matters more complicated, the current clinical guidelines and the paediatric neurology associations in the UK at the time of writing are quite negative about using medical cannabis, putting doctors in a very difficult position. Doctors rely on these clinical guidelines and physician society groups to guide their treatment decisions, and it can often be years before the evidence base in the research science impacts a guideline change. The lack of doctors willing to prescribe cannabis is another factor that inflates the cost, since without bulk supply and demand, the cost per patient is extremely high. Doctors often cite concern over possible unknown side effects, especially in children, despite the fact that side effects are usually rare and mild, while steroids and anti-seizure drugs have known serious side effects and are used without this same concern. As with all things around cannabis, research, education and removing stigmas are the way to overcome these fears.

Through my speaking and advocacy work in the UK, I have also met a brave teenager with epilepsy who was on so many drugs for his seizures he could not attend school and had zero quality of life. His desperation to be normal led to him trying black market cannabis oil after finding a patient medical cannabis information group online, as no doctor would help him get a prescription, even after the law change in November 2018 made it legal to do so. This had incredible results, bringing his seizures to almost nil and letting him reduce the other drugs drastically and come off some of them completely. He was able to return to school and feel like a normal teenager again. However, his medical team still refused to acknowledge that the near-miraculous change in his epilepsy had been due to the cannabis oil he was taking, and wouldn't help him access a legal prescription until there was 'more proof,' despite the good evidence *base that exists for CBD and epilepsy from the Epidiolex studies, as well as his case proof being right in front of them.*

Medical cannabis and CBD dosing

Advising on specific dosing and how to use medical cannabis and CBD for epilepsy is beyond the scope of this book, as it is a very serious condition that needs to be monitored closely by a doctor who understands both cannabis and epilepsy working alongside the main neurologist (epilepsy doctor) and the GP involved in the care of the patient. For educational purposes, however, I will discuss briefly some of the different cannabis medicine products that have been used clinically, dosage examples and types of cannabinoids that have shown benefits. Keep in mind that there are often large differences in dosages depending on the type of epilepsy, the age of the patient, other medications and a multitude of further factors.

Full-spectrum vs purified CBD

One of the things I have seen based on many individual cases is that using a full-spectrum high-CBD, low-THC cannabis oil seems to work better at reducing seizures than purified CBD on its own. This observation is supported by a recent study that looked at the data in those who had been treated with purified CBD vs used high-CBD medical cannabis oil in people with epilepsy, although the study had some methodology flaws to make a clear conclusion. This phenomenon I feel, along with many other experts, is likely due to the herbal synergy or entourage effect, when many different plant chemicals and cannabinoids in a full-extract oil work together to produce a greater effect on the disorder.[8] (See Chapter Five for a detailed discussion of CBD isolate vs full-spectrum.)

That being said, most of the published large-scale cannabinoid research studies in epilepsy have used pharma-grade purified CBD. The research on full-spectrum cannabis oils for epilepsy is still mainly from clinical experience and observational retrospective data collections and case studies. However, although results are not level 1 RCT (randomised controlled trial) evidence, they are too numerous and dramatic to be ignored. The effects of cannabis should be considered as evidence, especially in children whose condition has improved so dramatically in front of our eyes from starting these products when nothing else worked. It is a botanical medicine after all, and hard to fit into the narrow RCT box because it contains multiple cannabinoids in addition to CBD that may have anti-seizure activity.

Full-spectrum cannabis oil

Usually in epilepsy a high-CBD, low-THC cannabis oil or capsule by mouth is the main form of cannabis treatment tried by patients, since it has a longer duration of effect than inhaled vaporised cannabis (and vaporising is obviously not advisable in children). The 'start low, go slow' approach still applies to epilepsy dosing, especially in children, but the optimal dose on average will be much higher than other indications for using medical cannabis, such as for chronic pain, and hundreds of mg per day are often needed, even in kids.

In some patients who may stop responding well after a long time on the same high-CBD oil, another cannabinoid called THCA is sometimes added in a very small amount to the oil. Although THCA has far less published evidence for anti-seizure activity, in four published case reports[9] it has been helpful in very small doses of between 0.1 and 1mg/kg/day for seizure control used in combination with anti-seizure drugs. I have found this to be true clinically as well in those whose response to CBD starts to wane over time. THCA is generally not intoxicating and appears quite safe. The main issue with it is that it is hard to get. It degrades easily in the bottle with any heat or light exposure to active THC. I have used it clinically in Canada from a few suppliers of medical cannabis who make THCA oil specifically. So far in the UK it is rarely available outside of a made-to-order personalised product for a single patient, but I expect this will change. Despite a popular myth to the contrary, once THCA is taken orally as an oil or capsule it does not convert into THC in the body or cause intoxication.

In some cases, a small dose of THC oil is added to the CBD and THCA mix, still keeping the ratio of CBD to THC very high. This is done in cases where the response to CBD starts to wane over time, especially if THCA cannot be obtained. Doses are kept usually quite small and may lead to additional benefit, according to case reports clinically and preliminary published research.[10]

Cannabis oil reported dosage ranges in epilepsy

The dose of high-CBD medical cannabis that is effective in epilepsy varies widely. Most of the dosing being used on patients is based on unpublished clinical observations discovered using the 'start low, go slow' approach, as well as a very small amount of published research as a starting point or guide. The doses of CBD, for example, can range between 1 mg/kg/day and 7 mg/kg/day and also depend on whether cannabis is being used alongside other anti-epilepsy drugs for combined effect. The published doses for purified CBD only found that a dose of 20 mg/kg/day was effective for 120 children with a specific type of epilepsy called Dravet syndrome vs a placebo.[11]

Charlotte's story

Charlotte Figi is a young girl with Dravet syndrome. After multiple drugs had failed to treat her seizures (she was experiencing over 50 a day), her mother did a trial of high-CBD cannabis oil. When she added the oil in the right dose, the seizures were reduced to only 2–3 per month, and Charlotte's autistic self-injury behaviours also improved remarkably. Her dose sweet spot seemed to be 4 mg/kg/day; the results of the cannabis started to wear off and her seizures came back when she got down to 2 mg/kg/day and lower. This doesn't mean the same dose will work for other children, as each person may be slightly different, even with the same type of epilepsy. This was one of the earliest modern medicine cases of cannabis oil being used in a child with seizures, and the strain they used became known widely as Charlotte's Web.[12]

Drug/herb interactions

Among epilepsy drugs, clobazam has the most well-known interaction with cannabis. Although they can, under medical supervision, be used together, CBD in higher doses can elevate the level of clobazam in the bloodstream. At least in theory, other drug interactions are also possible, and a few case reports have indicated these with a drug called valproate. Drugs that affect blood clotting may also interact with CBD and cannabis (see Chapter Six for details of all drug/herb interactions). That is why close drug monitoring with a doctor is very important when using medical cannabis in the treatment of epilepsy. This is not an appropriate situation for self-experimentation.[13, 14]

Decreased response to therapy over time

Sometimes after someone has responded well initially to very high-CBD, minimal-THC oil for their seizures, it can happen that they become less responsive again. The exact reasons behind this are not known, but there are various potential factors that likely play a role, including:

- Batch-to-batch variation in the minor cannabinoids in the oil that may be contributing to the anti-seizure effect.
- Changes in endocannabinoid and other receptors. This theory comes from several cases (one of which I have been involved with personally) where a 'washout' period from cannabis and CBD was done under close supervision which may 'reset' the response level. When the cannabis and CBD were restarted at a lower dose, the response improved again. The risk is that in the washout period, more seizures could occur, which is why doing this under very close medical supervision in a controlled environment is recommended.

For additional information, see references[15, 16, 17].

CONCLUSION

I hope these pages have been able to dispel the many myths surrounding the cannabis plant, and cut through the confusion about CBD and medical cannabis. Far from being the dangerous drug we grew up hearing about, cannabis has much to offer us. It has huge potential for medicine, as well as helping us all to just cope better with the stresses and pressures of modern life. We still have a lot to learn about how cannabis and CBD work in our bodies and brains, but as the hundreds of research studies referenced in this book, as well as my clinical experience, shows, we are getting there.

Even if you are reading this as someone I'd call 'canna-curious', but decide not to take it yourself, I hope you are now armed with the knowledge to speak confidently about cannabis and CBD to your doctor, your neighbour, your children or your grandmother. The latest research has unburdened cannabis of any stigma that was once attached to it, giving us solid evidence and allowing us to reclaim it as is a tool that is there should you or your loved ones need it in the future.

If you plan to take CBD or cannabis, I trust that you now know where you can start, how to pick a good CBD product and how to investigate whether medical cannabis may be something worth exploring with your doctor.

Plants were the first medicine humans learned to use. Despite all the amazing high-tech advances we have courtesy of modern drug science, plant medicines have not become obsolete. Quite the opposite. They are beginning a renaissance of sorts thanks to a collective yearning for more natural approaches to common health and wellness concerns.

The golden era of believing we were very close to having single pharmaceutical drugs able to cure every condition is over. Many modern drugs have failed to offer the hope and relief people were anticipating. This is especially true for complicated conditions like chronic pain, mental health and stress-related issues, which are reaching epidemic proportions. Our bodies are not machines that can be simply broken down into parts that can be easily fixed with a single drug. Instead, we are complex, dynamic beings, which is why whole-plant medicines seem to work so well with our biochemistry. Hundreds of different active ingredients in a single plant medicine interact and work in synergy with our brain and body on many diverse biochemical pathways, a feat that would be impossible for a single drug.

I see the interest in cannabis as part of a bigger shift in medicine towards more open-minded holistic thinking, more inclusive of non-pharma-drug healing modalities and more prepared to study alternative remedies to increase the evidence base and our understanding of how they work. This is medicine that involves a partnership between doctors and patients; that empowers us and gets us back in tune with our bodies rather than disconnecting us; that is based in evidence but finds that evidence in a broader context than what can be easily tested in a narrow drug-development funnel style of research. It isn't Eastern or Western, conventional or alternative, ancient or modern, but simply good medicine.

REFERENCES

For a list of resources by chapter,
please go to www.drdanigordon.com/cbd-bible-references

ACKNOWLEDGEMENTS

This work would not be possible without my patients and clients who have been my greatest teachers over the years, bravely sharing their stories and partnering with me as we went on this journey together. A massive thanks to my most wonderful colleagues Dr Ron Reznick and Dr Ron Puhkey for their friendship and mentorship in family and integrative medicine over the years and for giving me the privilege of being a part of their practice; and to Jean Southgate for her enduring support, friendship and patience with my unending mail.

I also owe a debt of gratitude to the many brilliant scientists and medical colleagues on multiple continents who have pioneered cannabis as a medicine and contributed immensely to my own knowledge about the plant with their years of research studies and by sharing their tips on how to use it clinically, especially Dr Ethan Russo, Dr Roger Pertwee, Arno Hazekamp and Dr Scott Shannon. A big thanks to my fellow cannabis medicine docs around the world, especially Dr Sandra Carrillo for her support and collegiality across continents and my amazing colleagues who have become dear friends working on cannabis in the UK, Dr Lili Galindo, Dr Chloe Sakal, Dr Leon Barron, Dr Callie Seaman, Professor Mike Barnes and last but certainly not least Professor David Nutt, who has been an inspiration and a leading light in drug research and policy reform.

I owe much of the success of this book and my work in medical cannabis to my husband Nick. His unwavering support and encouragement over the years has given me the courage to pursue integrative medicine and cannabis medicine to help my patients, especially in the early days before it gained larger mainstream medicine support and understanding.

Thanks to my family for their support along this journey, with its many uncertainties, and especially to my parents for always encouraging and supporting my slightly unconventional medical career, and my mum-in-law Chris, who has supported me in untold ways over the years.

I want to thank the many patient advocates I have had the pleasure of working with and getting to know personally, including the inspirational Hannah Deacon, Carly Barton, Talin Sellian, Callie Blackwell, Lucy Stafford, Charlotte Caldwell, Peter Carroll and the many more who work tirelessly for the rights and health of patients.

Thank you to my amazing agent extraordinaire Rachel Mills and my international agent Alexandra Cliff for being the best team any author could ever ask for.

I owe a massive thanks to my UK editor Pippa Wright (nickname on my speed dial: Editing Guru) for her patience, humour and brilliance working on this manuscript, and to my amazing team at Orion Spring, who have gone above and beyond and been an author's dream to work with. In the US, a massive thanks to my editors Haley Weaver, Beth deGuzman and the team from Grand Central Hachette USA for believing in this book and helping me get it out there in my integrative medicine home. On the Canadian side, a huge thanks to my editor Brad Wilson and his team from HarperCollins Canada for trusting me and this book to tackle the huge need for more information and education about cannabis and CBD, which is now widely available but still often misunderstood, and for helping me to reach my fellow Canadians in the country where my journey with medical cannabis started. In Spain, a huge thank you to my translation and publishing team Carlos Ramos and Blanca Rosa Roca at Roca Editorial; and in Poland to my Polish editor Małgorzata Święcicka and Piotr Wawrzeńczyk at Booklab Agency (you have made me and my 96-year-old Polish grandad proud to have this in Polish!).

ABOUT THE AUTHOR

Dr Dani Gordon is a Canadian and American board-certified medical doctor, writer, speaker and published researcher. She completed her family medicine residency at the University of British Columbia and went on to become an American board-qualified specialist in integrative medicine, the newest American physician sub-specialty of conventional medicine.

In her Canadian medical practice she was one of the early adopters of cannabis medicine, treating thousands of patients with medical cannabis in an integrative chronic disease referral practice.

She trained the first UK physicians in cannabis medicine, consults for government groups, companies and international organisations on cannabis and is a founding member and current vice chair of the UK Medical Cannabis Clinicians Society (MCCS).

She is also a leading wellness expert specialising in holistic mental health, peak mental performance, stress resilience and burnout recovery, and has studied meditation, yoga and natural medicine extensively throughout India and South East Asia with traditional teachers.

She has been featured in numerous publications, including *Vogue*, *Forbes*, the *Sunday Times* and the *Guardian*, and has appeared on the BBC and Channel 4.

She now lives in London with her husband Nick and their dog Indica (Indy) the Cavapoo.

INDEX